M000205984

CHAKRAS HEALING FOR BEGINNERS

Discovering the Secrets to Detect and
Dissolve Energy Blockages - Balance and
Awaken your full Potential through
Yoga, Meditation and Mindfulness

By

Sarah Allen

© Copyright 2020 by Sarah Allen all rights reserved.

This document is geared towards providing exact and reliable information about the topic and issue covered. The publication is sold with the idea that the publisher is not required to render accounting, officially permitted, or otherwise qualified services. If advice is necessary, legal or professional, a practiced individual in the profession should be ordered.

From a Declaration of Principles which was accepted and approved equally by a Committee of the American Bar Association and a Committee of Publishers and Associations.

In no way is it legal to reproduce, duplicate, or transmit any part of this document in either electronic means or printed format. Recording of this publication is strictly prohibited, and any storage of this document is not allowed unless with written permission from the publisher. All rights reserved.

The information provided herein is stated to be truthful and consistent, in that any liability, in terms of inattention or otherwise, by any usage or abuse of any policies, processes, or directions contained within is the solitary and utter responsibility of the recipient reader. Under no circumstances will any legal responsibility or blame be held against the publisher for any reparation, damages, or monetary loss due to the information herein, either directly or indirectly.

Respective authors own all copyrights not held by the publisher.

The information herein is offered for informational purposes solely and is universal as so.

The presentation of the information is without a contract or any guarantee assurance.

The trademarks that are used are without any consent, and the publication of the trademark is without permission or backing by the trademark owner. All trademarks and brands within this book are for clarifying purposes only and are owned by the owners themselves, not affiliated with this document.

TABLE OF CONTENTS

CHAPTER 1

WHAT ARE THEY AND WHAT ARE THEY FOR?

The chakras are points of energy that, when in balance, enhance our vital energy. In turn, that energy assures us of greater well-being both physically and mentally. In recent years, a wide variety of complementary therapies of oriental origin have become popular in the West, recognized for their ability to promote well-being. While the evidence on their safety and efficacy is limited, the testimonies of those who have tried them have aroused the interest of many patients. This time, we want to talk a little more about the chakras and their uses.

According to sources such as Wikipedia, the chakras come from Hinduism and refer to centers of immeasurable energy located in the body, specifically from the perineum to the area of the aura that is above the crown. There are seven, according to the Hindu tradition, and each one has a determined, energetic vibration that is associated with aspects of life and health. Let's see more about this.

What are the chakras, and how do they work?

The term chakra comes from Sanskrit and means "circle" or "disk." According to Hinduism, the chakras are 7 energy centers that are located in different parts of the human body. They function as "valves," regulating the flow of energy and, depending on their location, vary in their vibratory force and speed.

In India, it is believed that inhaled air (known as prana energy) runs through the body giving strength to the energy centers. The chakras receive, accumulate and distribute prana to optimize the functions of various parts of our body.

Therefore, since ancient times, they have been used as a resource in energy medicine, suggesting that they can contribute to treating certain medical conditions and problems.

However, although studies have been carried out in this regard, such as a study published recently in Global Advances in Health and Medicine, there is insufficient evidence to ensure that they are useful against diseases.

According to this research, the chakra system is related to the endocrine system of the body. In addition, as we have already mentioned, it has 7 vital energy centers, which mainly focus on the spine.

Being producers of energy vortices, the chakras, when healthy, provide energy information through which the body's systems create a global information system, which will be the one that affects well-being. However, more research is required to determine if these types of therapies really help to fight diseases through the subtle energy generated at these points.

What feelings are the chakras associated with?

Despite the lack of evidence, chakras continue to stand out in alternative medicine as an adjunct against problems related to the mentioned glands. In addition, following the Hindu and Buddhist texts that speak about it, they are also associated with certain feelings.

1. Muladhara the root chakra

- It is located between the anus and the genitals.
- The color that identifies it is red.
- Its element is the earth.
- It is blocked by fear. Therefore, let the fears be clearly displayed to free them.

11

2. Svadhisthana o chakra Sacro

- It is found in the sacrum.
- It is associated with the color orange.
- Its assigned element is water.
- Guilt blocks it. Hence, we have to get rid of this. And, for this, it is necessary to know how to forgive.

3. Manipura or solar plexus chakra

- It is located two fingers above the navel.
- Its color is yellow.
- Fire is its element.
- It is blocked by shame.

4. Anahata or heart chakra

- It is located in the heart region.
- Its color is green.
- Its assigned element is air.
- It is blocked by pain.
- It is related to the feelings of the heart.

5. Vishuddha o chakra de la Garganta

- It is located in the throat region.
- It corresponds to the color blue.
- Its element is ether.
- It is related to communication.

6. Ajna or third eye chakra

- It is located between the two eyes.
- Its color is violet.
- It is associated with intuition and taste.
- It is blocked by illusion.

7. Sahasrara or crown chakra

- It is in the crown.
- It corresponds to the color violet or indigo.
- It is blocked by worldly ties.

The chakras are another resource that give us oriental medicine as a supplement to promote wellness. However, given the lack of evidence, it is important to consider it a therapeutic option and not a first-line treatment against diseases.

To learn more about its benefits and practice, it is convenient to seek the guidance of an expert. It is often combined with other health therapies, such as yoga, quartz baths, and deep breathing exercises.

CHAPTER 2

7 WONDERFUL ENERGY CENTERS

The chakras are energy centers located in the human body that have been identified by oriental culture. In these points, biological and psychological aspects of our way of relating are integrated, so that through its balance we can achieve well-being.

According to Hinduism, the balance of the chakras is achieved based on how we interact with ourselves, with other people, with nature, and with the divine. Being unbalanced is when some personal and social dysfunctions manifest.

It is important to know that each of the chakras is related to a color, a location in the body, and a sound, which promotes their balance and activation when meditating. Here we tell you about each of these wonderful energy centers.

"Nothing leaves our life until it teaches us what we need to learn."

-Pema Chödrön-

First chakra: root chakra

Name: Muladhara

Color: Red

Associated element: Earth

Location: The base of the column

Sound: LAM

This chakra is related to biological, psychological, and relational support. In this way, this center has to do with group strength and roots. The associated parts of our body are the legs, the feet, the immune system, the spine, and the bones.

In addition, this energy center is the first one we develop and is the one that sustains everyone else. Through this, we develop in relationships with nature, with others and with ourselves. In addition, it is strongly connected with the energy of our ancestors, which can help us in the most difficult moments.

However, on a psychological level, it has to do with security, defense and the ability to provide needs. These aspects foster support, as they have to do with the strength, protection, learning and beliefs of our groups.

15

When this chakra is not in equilibrium, it could be associated with dysfunctions from a lack of support. For example, immune system conditions, back pain, and leg pain. And on a psychological level, it can be related to mood disorders such as depression and anxiety.

To keep it in balance, we must be aware of the way we relate to our roots, for example, the way we are with our families and the beliefs we have learned. In addition, we can be in balance through meditation.

«Your beliefs are not made of realities. It is your reality that is made of beliefs».

-Richard Bandler-

Chakra 2: the wonderful way in which we interact!

Name: Svadhisthana

Color: Orange

Associated element: Water

Location: From the lower abdomen to the navel area

Sound: Vam

It's about the dynamics we have with others, with nature and with ourselves. Therefore, it has to do with the vision we have of the world. Thus, it is linked to creativity, money management, ethics and sexuality. In other words, it relates to the way we link and interact.

Now, in our body, it is mainly in: the sexual organs, the intestine, the bladder and the vertebrae. Thus, dysfunctions are associated with problems in these places. On a psychological level, the imbalance reflects aspects such as: attachment, pressure, lack of satisfaction, impulsivity, and a feeling that the world is flat.

To keep it in balance we can be attentive to our creative selves, the way we manage money, the ability to put ourselves in the place of others and the way in which we communicate. To activate it, meditation is useful.

Chakra 3: personal power!

Name: Manipuraka

Color: Yellow

Associated item: Fire

Location: Solar plexus

Sound: RAM

It is the chakra of self-esteem; it is related to intention, coordination and control. This chakra has to do with our self and with our personality.

The associated organs are: the stomach, the liver, the kidneys, the pancreas, the adrenal glands, and the central part of the spine. When not in balance, they manifest: fear, intimidation, anorexia or bulimia, arthritis and chronic or acute indigestion, among others.

As for the emotional manifestations, this is one of the chakras that is linked to: trust, self-care, and others, and responsibility when making decisions. When it is in imbalance we have problems in these aspects. To balance it, meditation is useful, to connect with our inner strength and visualize what we truly want.

"The measure of what we are is what we do with what we have."

-Vince Lombardi-

Chakra 4: the incredible power of emotions

Name: Anahata

Color: Green

Associated item: Air

Location: Chest center

Sound: Yam

This is the energy center of unconditional love. It is related to understanding, love and forgiveness. On an organic level it has to do with: the heart, lungs, shoulders, arms, circulatory system and diaphragm. Then, physical dysfunctions reflect: circulatory system failures, asthma, breast cancer, and pneumonia.

Its emotional manifestations are: love and hate, self-centeredness, loneliness, commitment, forgiveness, compassion, hope and trust. Thus, emotional dysfunctions have to do with: dependence, confusion, not believing, lack of trust, and inability to forgive and commit.

«Love unconditionally, don't ask for anything in return. You will receive a lot without asking - you will make it something else - but don't be a beggar. In love to be an emperor. Just give and wait, what happens: you will receive a thousand times more ».

-Osho-

Chakra 5: the will

Name: Vishudda

Color: Blue

Associated Element: Ether

Location: Throat

Sound: Ham

Chakra 5 is that of will and self-expression. The organs involved in this energy center are: the throat, the thyroid, the trachea, the cervical vertebrae, the mouth, the hypothalamus, the teeth, and the gums, among others. Physical dysfunctions have to do with conditions in these parts, for example: hoarseness or thyroid disorders.

Emotionally it is related to: choice, expression, faith, knowledge, judgment, criticism, addiction and following goals. Then, it is linked to the ability to express what we feel, make decisions and follow motivations. When it is unbalanced it has to do with the way of judging and the difficulty in communicating and deciding.

"Who has will has strength."

-Menandro-

Chakra 6: the power of our mind

Name: Ajna

Color: Violet

Associated item: Light

Location: The center of the forehead

Sound: Om

This wonderful center of energy is the one that connects with wisdom, intuition and perception. On a physical level it is related to: the nervous system, eyes, ears and nose. In imbalance there may be dysfunctions such as: neurological disorders, blindness, deafness and learning problems.

Now, it is manifested psychologically in: the way to evaluate ourselves, the truth, emotional intelligence and tolerance when listening to other people's ideas. In other words, it is the power we have to evaluate our own beliefs and attitudes, introspection and the capacity for judgment. If it is in imbalance we show problems in these aspects.

"Rejoice because every place is here and every moment is now."

-Buddha-

Chakra 7: the spiritual connection

Name: Sahasrara

Color: White

Associated item: Cosmic sound

Location: Crown

Sound: Silence

This is the energy center of the spiritual, of the transcendent, the force chakra between mind, body and spirit. So, it is related to: the ability we have to trust life, generosity, global vision, faith, inspiration, and devotion. When it is not balanced, energy disorders and extreme sensitivity to environmental factors can occur.

«The secret of human freedom is to act well, without attachment to the results».

-Bhagavad Gita-

Now, as you have seen, to revitalize our chakras we could meditate and thus enter into a deep connection. Also, to facilitate the practice and balance of the chakras, we can focus on the colors, sounds, elements and places of the body of each chakra. In addition, it will also help us visualize the balance we want to reach into our lives and perform healthy practices emotionally and physically.

Furthermore, we can listen to our body and mind to know which chakras are in imbalance, and try to reach a state of fullness. It's about being attentive to the problems we have and trying to solve them. Meditation could help us connect and find a way out.

According to the oriental culture, peace is achieved through the care of this energy flow. It is a way that allows personal growth and from which you can learn step by step to reach harmony, through deep connection. In addition, being attentive to our chakras is a source of self-knowledge. Learn from yourself and your environment by seeking energy balance because, as Caroline Myers said, "the healing of the body comes through the healing of the soul."

Myss, C. (1996). Anatomy of the Spirit: The healing of the body comes through the soul. Pocket Zeta, Spain.

CHAPTER 3

THE CHAKRAS, ENERGY POINTS THAT YOU MUST ACTIVATE

Here we discuss how you can optimize the chakras in different ways: gems, aromas, music, massages, etc.

The chakras are 7 energy points that are strategically distributed in our body. They regulate our health. In addition, they can influence us emotionally and spiritually.

For this reason, if we do not lead a coherent, kind and beneficial lifestyle, we cannot find balance. We could even get blocked.

Next we will discuss how you can improve the functioning of the chakras. For this, we can resort to some natural methods such as music, aromas, gems, colors or massages.

So if you want to improve your day-to-day life and enjoy well-being, do not hesitate to give them a chance. Rest assured, it will be worth it.

As mentioned earlier, the chakras are 7 energy points that are found along our spine and head.

They follow a straight line right in the center of our body and regulate the different functions of the body, as well as our abilities and emotions. They are the following:

- Root Chakra: is located at the base of the spine. It is linked to trust.
- Sacral chakra: It is found in the sacrum bone, above the genitals. It is related to sexuality and creativity.
- Solar plexus chakra: the third chakra is two fingers above the navel. It is linked with wisdom.
- Heart chakra: it is in the center of the chest. Thus, this chakra is related to love and healing.
- Throat Chakra: This chakra corresponds to the throat and, therefore, also to the thyroid. Work communication.
- Eyebrow chakra: in the eyebrows we find the famous third eye, related to consciousness and knowledge.
- Chakra of the crown: in the crown is the seventh and last chakra. It is the energetic center of spirituality, which connects our body with the highest.

1. Musical notes

To begin, we must know that the chakras correspond to the 7 musical notes. It is not a coincidence, since everything in nature has its harmony.

Therefore, music can also help us physically and spiritually. And we will start, for example, singing the note of the chakra that we want to help balance. Thus, each chakra corresponds to its note:

- Root: Do
- Sacral: Re
- Solar Plexus: Mi
- Heart: Fa
- Throat: Sun
- Entree: The
- Crown: Yes

2. Essential oils

Aromatherapy can offer us a pleasant and delicious therapy by means of essential oils. Thus, it can help us improve our physical, spiritual and emotional well-being. In this way, each chakra has its specific aromas:

- **Root:** cedar and clove
- **Sacral:** ylang-ylang and sandalwood
- **Solar plexus:** lavender, rosemary and bergamot

- **Heart:** rose, mint and musk
- **Throat:** sage and eucalyptus
- **Entree:** mint and jasmine
- **Crown**: olive and lotus

First, we can use the essential oils to massage the corresponding points.

However, we must ensure that they are of the highest quality, since there are many chemical essences on the market. These only work to give a scent, but not to cure.

3. Colors

The chakras are related to different types of vibrations which, in turn, correspond to colors.

In this sense, the chromotherapy or healing through color can help us in finding balance.

Therefore, the chakras correspond to the following colors:

- Root: Red
- Sacral: Orange
- Solar Plexus: Yellow
- Heart: Green
- Throat: Blue

- Entrecejo: Indigo
- Crown: Violet

The colors that surround us can influence our quality of life.

Actually, when choosing clothes or accessories, painting the house or putting certain pictures, we are promoting one aspect or the other.

For this reason, it is recommended that you choose them conscientiously. In addition, you can also use chromotherapy lamps.

4. Gems

Gemmotherapy is a curative therapy according to which each gem or stone would have medicinal properties.

Also, each chakra has its own. In this way, we can put it on that part of the body through accessories or while we are resting. In this sense, the corresponding gems are the following:

- **Root:** Ruby and Garnet
- **Sacral:** amber and topaz
- **Solar Plexus:** Agate
- **Heart:** rose quartz and malachite

- **Throat:** aquamarine, turquoise and lapis lazuli
- **Entrecejo:** amethyst and moonstone
- **Crown:** white quartz and diamond

5. Massages

Finally, massages can also contribute to improving the functioning of our body's energy points.

Thus, there are different therapies such as yoga or reiki that work with this type of energy. However, we must perform them in appropriate places and with certified professionals.

In addition, we can combine massages with the other techniques to multiply their effects.

Some examples are massages with essential oils and gems, set with colored light and with the appropriate musical accompaniment. An experience for all the senses and levels of the individual!

CHAPTER 4

THE MISSION AND FUNCTIONING OF THE CHAKRAS

In this chapter, we will look at the most fundamental information on the functioning of the chakras. The theoretical understanding of these relationships is the basis on which practical knowledge about each of the individual chakras described in this book is based.

The writings that tradition has bequeathed to us mention a large number of chakras: 88,000. This means that in the human body there is hardly any point other than a sensitive organ for the reception, transformation and retransmission of energies. However, most of these chakras are very small and play a subordinate role in the energy system. There are approximately 40 secondary chakras that are assigned greater importance. The most important of these are in the area of the spleen, in the nape of the neck, in the palms of the hands and on the soles of the feet. The seven main chakras, located along a vertical axis next to the anterior half of the body, are so decisive for the functioning of the most fundamental and essential areas of the body, spirit and soul of man, that a chapter has been dedicated to each of them. In these chapters you will be able to see what specific mood-spiritual qualities are related to each of the chakras, which body areas are subject to their influence, how the blockages of each of the chakras affect, and many other things.

Here, let's describe the characteristics that are common to the seven main chakras. They truly settle in man's etheric body. They resemble funnel-shaped floral calyxes and a varied number of petals. Therefore, in the cultural sphere of the East they are often also called parrot flowers. The subdivisions of the flowers into independent petals represent the nadis or energy channels through which energies flow and penetrate the chakras and through which energy is relayed from the chakras to the non-material bodies. Its number varies from four channels in the radical center to almost a thousand energy channels in the center of the crown.

The chakras are in a permanent circular motion. To this quality they owe the name "chakra," which in Sanskrit means "wheel." The rotating movement of these wheels causes the energy to be drawn into the chakras. If the direction of rotation changes, the energy is radiated from the chakras.

The chakras can rotate to the right or to the left. Here one can recognize a contrasting principle in man and woman, or complementation in the expression of the energies of different "species" since the same chakras that in man turn to the right (clockwise), in the woman turn left, and vice versa. Every right turn has as its peculiarity a predominance of the male quality, an accentuation of the yang according to Chinese doctrine; that is, it represents will and activity, and in its negative form of manifestation, also aggression and violence. Every left turn has a predominance of yin and represents sensitivity and agreement, and in its negative aspect, weakness.

The direction of rotation changes from one chakra to another. Thus, the basal chakra of man turns to the right, and more actively expresses the qualities of this center: in the sense of conquest and dominance in the material and sexual realm. On the other hand, the woman's first chakra has a sense of rotation to the left, which makes her more sensitive to the earth's life-giving and spawning force, which flows through the radical center. In the second chakra the signs are reversed: the direction of rotation to the right in the woman indicates greater active energy in the expression of feelings; man's sense of rotation to the left can preferably be interpreted here as the receptive, often even as a passive attitude. And so on.

Sense of spin of chakras in women

The continuous line that rises undulating symbolizes Pingala, solar energy, and the dotted line represents Ida, the lunar force.

Knowing the direction of rotation of the chakras allows them to be incorporated into some forms of therapy. For example, in aromatherapy you can apply the aromas with a circular movement in the corresponding direction, or also a plot with the precious stones turns in the same sense that the energy centers have.

Most people's chakras have an average length of approximately 10 centimeters. In each of the energy centers there are all the chromatic vibrations, although it always masters a certain color, which coincides with the main function of the corresponding chakra. In a superior development of man, the chakras continue to spread and increase their vibration frequency. Also, their colors become lighter and more radiant.

The size and number of vibrations (frequency) of the chakras determine the quantity and quality of the energies they absorb from the most varied sources. These are energies that come to us from the cosmos, the stars, nature, the radiation of all things and all the people of our environment, our different non-material bodies, and also from the original unmanifested reason of all beings. These energies reach the chakras, in part, through the nadis, and, in part, flow into them directly. The two most important and fundamental forms of energy are absorbed through the radical center and the coronal center. Between these two chakras runs the Sushumna, to which all the energy centers are attached through their "petioles" and which feeds all of them with life force. It is the channel through which the so-called Kundalini energy rises, which rests, "rolled like a snake", at the lower end of the spine, and whose gateway is the radical center. Kundalini energy represents the cosmic energy of creation, which in Indian wisdom is also called Shakti or the female manifestation of God. This active aspect of the divine being provokes all manifestations of creation. Its opposite pole is the pure, amorphous and self-inherent aspect of the divine being, in which we will have a closer look later.

In most people, Kundalini energy only flows through Sushumna in scant proportion. As he wakes up from a growing development of consciousness, he ascends through the spinal canal in an ever-increasing flow, and activating the different chakras. This activation results in an extension of the energy centers and an acceleration of their frequencies. Kundalini energy feeds chakras with the energy vibration that empowers men to gradually open up in the course of their evolution all the faculties and energies that act in the different energy planes and materials of creation, with the intention to integrate these energies into your life.

During its ascent, Kundalini energy is transformed into a different vibration in each chakra, corresponding to the functions of the respective chakra. This vibration is minimal in the radical center and finds its maximum expression in the coronal center. Transformed vibrations are relayed to different non-material bodies or to the physical body, and perceived as feelings, ideas and physical sensations.

The degree to which a person allows the action of Kundalini energy depends on the degree of consciousness he has in the different spheres of life represented by the chakras, and the extent to which stress and unprocessed experiences have caused blockages in the chakras. The more conscious a person is, the more open and active their chakras are, so that Kundalini energy can flow to them more intensely; and the more intense this flow of energy, the more active the chakras become, which in turn awakens greater awareness. In this way a permanent cycle of mutual influence arises, as soon as we begin to eliminate our blockages and to walk a path of the development of consciousness.

In addition to Kundalini energy, there is another force flowing into each of the chakras through the Sushumna canal of the spine. It is the energy of the pure divine being, of the unmanifested aspect of God. It enters through the coronal chakra and makes man know in all planes of life the amorphous existential aspect of God as the original, immutable and penetrating reason of that manifestation. This energy is particularly suitable for removing chakra blockages. In Indian wisdom it is called Shiva, the divinity, which is the great destroyer of ignorance and which, with its mere presence, unleashes a transformation towards the divine.

This representation of chakras from Nepal is approximately 350 years old. The seven main chakras, represented by parrot flowers, can be recognized. Each of these chakra flowers represents a plane of consciousness, starting with the lower ones and ending with the upper ones at the top. The main energy channels, Sushumna, Ida and Pingala, can also be recognized.

Thus, Shiva and Shakti work hand in hand in the integral development of the person, which we have integrated into our lives both the divine and all the planes of the relative being.

Alongside Sushumna, there are two other energy channels that play a particularly important role in the energy system: in Sanskrit they are called Ida and Pingala. Pingala doubles as a carrier of solar energy, full of burning and motor force. This channel starts to the right of the radical chakra and ends at the top of the right nostril. Ida is the carrier of the cooling and serene lunar energy. This channel begins to the left of the radical chakra and ends in the left nostril. On their way from the radical center to the nose, both nadis sink around Sushumna.

Ida and Pingala have the ability to absorb prana directly from the air by breathing, and to expel poisonous substances into the exhalation. Together with Sushumna, they constitute the three main channels of the energy system. In addition, there are a large number of other nadis that provide chakras with energies from secondary chakras and non-material bodies, and that relay that energy to neighboring energy bodies.

But chakras also directly absorb vibrations from the environment, vibrations that correspond to their frequencies. Thus, through their different forms of operation, they unite us with the events of our environment, nature and the universe, serving as antennas for the full range of energy vibrations. We can also call chakras non-material sensory organs. Our physical body, together with its senses, is a vehicle adapted to the laws of life of our planet. And with whose help we manage in the external realm of life, but with which we can simultaneously realize our values on earth, and know internal processes. The chakras serve as receptors for all the energy vibrations and information that come from the physical realm. They are the openings that unite us with the unlimited world of the most subtle energies.

The chakras also radiate energy directly into the environment, thus modifying the atmosphere around us. Through the chakras we can emit healing vibrations and messages, conscious and unconscious, influencing both positively and negatively on people, situations and even matter.

To experience an inner fulness, and the energy, creativity, knowledge, love and blessing associated with it, all chakras must be open and work in mutual harmony. However, this circumstance occurs in very few people. In general, different chakras have a different degree of activation. And many times only the lower two chakras are activated. In people who hold an outstanding social position, or who in some way exert a great influence, it is common that, in addition, the solar plexus chakra is disproportionately active. Any combination of open, blocked or marked chakras may exist in a particular sense. In addition, these degrees oscillate throughout a lifetime, since at different times different topics may become important.

Therefore, the knowledge of the chakras can provide you with invaluable help for self-knowledge, and guide you on your way to discover all the innate faculties, giving you a life of maximum fullness and joy.

Cycles of human evolution in light of chakra theory

In our universe, everything is subject to clearly specific rhythms and cycles. These begin on the atomic plane and extend to all forms of existence of the entire creation. In a heartbeat and in our breathing, in the rhythmic succession of days and nights, in the seasons, and even in the predictable displacement of the stars, we detect the rhythmic regularities described. Also in the evolution of living beings we can detect periodic cycles. Thus, for example, in the plants, we observe how the germ first appears, then the leaves, the bud, the flower, and finally the fruit. A certain sequence of evolutionary phases is always respected, which are not freely interchangeable with each other: it is quite evident that man, as being intelligent in a material body, has also evolved according to periodic laws. Not only do they get older every day and their abilities and experiences increase, but their evolution is consumed in very special mental and spiritual evolutionary cycles. Not all the issues are of the same importance in all times of life, and if we look at this fact more closely we realize that "Mother Nature" gives us very specific tasks in specific times, tasks that must be solved at that exact time. While these tasks can be presented with different 'clothes,' it can generally be said that a given evolution can only be optimally summed up at a certain time in life. For example, it is very difficult to recover at 25 years of age, an evolution that we omitted when we were between 5 and 12 years old. And so it happens that the vital building of some people is supported for a lifetime on wobbly foundations, because in the years of youth certain experiences were not made or only certain capacities were insufficiently formed.

The knowledge of the cycles of life is not new: in any case we could say that it has been lost again. Various intellectual schools, however, continue to imply this knowledge today with the total evolution of man. In anthroposophical circles, and within them Waldorf's pedagogy is fundamentally known, these relationships are well known. Learning plans were reasonably developed to adapt them to a correct human evolution based on evolutionary cycles of children's natural and internal processes. The founder of the anthroposophical movement, Rudolf Steiner, left us an immense legacy on this subject (for example, the book Vom Lebenslauf des Menschen "The Curriculum of Man"). In anthroposophical anthropology we recognize a vital path that takes place in clearly articulated rhythmic phases, divided into "seven-year cycles." It is quite clear that time hides in itself different qualities, or that at certain times in his life man is differently "open" to certain influences and experiences, and therefore "mature" for totally specific evolutionary progress.

It is interesting that this knowledge is seamlessly integrated into the knowledge of the functioning and functions of our chakra system. Thus, starting from the basal center, we move every seven years to a different chakra, whose qualities constitute a fundamental theme of our life during that time. Simultaneously, this period is divided into seven additional main themes, each of them lasting one year, and they also begin in the basal chakra, to travel year after year one of the following seven chakras.

Then begins a new cycle of another seven years, but this time with the fundamental pattern of the second chakra. Thus, year after year we go through one more evolutionary stage, which consists of the fundamental theme of the septenary and seven main themes of a year. After 5 x 7 years we have reached about half of our life. After 7 x 7 years of life we have finished a full cycle of 49 years. So as we enter the fiftieth year of life, a whole new stage begins, we effectively have the opportunity to start again from the beginning, but this time in a "top octave" of evolution. Also after the age of 50, totally special learning stages await us, which must be summed up. Thus, some people end at the age of 98, the second great journey through human evolutionary cycles.

Every year that passes brings us a new main theme, and every seven years a new fundamental theme; in this process the topics are always complimented in the most optimal way. The knowledge of the meaning and function of each chakra shows us the way to optimally take advantage of each particular year for the benefit of our evolution. In addition, it allows us to understand in greater depth the evolution of our children and always give them the right kind of dedication and stimuli that will be most valuable to them in a given time.

Also, in the material plane, a transformation is consuming with a cyclical rhythm of seven years. You may have already heard the existence of the biological proof that our bodies are completely renewed every seven years. At seven years old, all body cells have been replaced by new ones, and we are completely new people from a physical point of view. If, on the other hand, on the psychic plane it seems as if in those seven years nothing has actually changed, it is because our emotional body is loaded with patterns similar to those of the beginning of this period of time. But it can also happen that after a long time you meet again with a person who has taken a violent evolutionary step. A fundamental change is absolutely possible in seven years.

In the following pages we will try to convey an overview about the experiences that man must broadly navigate in each of his years of life, and the influences to which he is particularly sensitive. In the next chapter we will explain in more detail some examples.

CHAPTER 5

THE ORIGIN OF BLOCKAGES IN CHAKRAS

By our true nature, we are one with that strength that manifests itself in the vibrations and regular laws infinitely varied, in the colors and shapes, in the aromas and sounds of all creation. We're not separated from anything. The most intimate core of our being lives in inseparable communion with the absolute, immutable, omnipresent being that we call God and which has produced and penetrates all areas of relative existence. This pure, unlimited existence is by nature the glory.

As soon as the silent and calm ocean of the divine being is curled in waves of joy, the dance of creation begins, of which we too are a form of manifestation and in which we can participate, in all its planes, through our bodies, not necessarily the physical body.

However, we lose consciousness of unity at the moment when we begin to rely exclusively on the information that comes to us through the physical senses and rational understanding, forgetting our origin and our divine base. We lost the feeling of inner fullness and safety in life and began to look for it in the outdoor field. But in that quest the coffering of full consummation was let down over and over again. This experience raised anguish over a new disappointment. We also forget that we can never be extinguished, since death only means a variation of the external form.

Anguish always causes a contraction and, therefore, a grip or blockage, which in turn intensifies the feeling of separation and allows the anguish to continue to grow. Breaking this vicious cycle and regaining lost unity is the declared goal of almost all the spiritual pathways of East and West.

Chakras are those connection points in man's energy system in which blockages conditioned by distress are preferably established. There may also be other locks along the nadis. When these contractions become permanent, they cause vital energies not to flow freely and feed our various bodies with everything they need to reflect and maintain the awareness of unity. When the experience of separation, abandonment, inner emptiness and fear of death prompts us to seek in the outside world what we can only find in the most intimate of our being, we become dependent on the love and recognition of other people of the sensory arrivals, success and material possession. Instead of enriching our lives,

45

these things become peremptory needs with which we try to fill the void. If we lose them, we suddenly find ourselves at nothingness, and the slight sense of anguish that accompanies almost everyone is presented to us again as real. And, of course, it is the others who take from us what we so evidently need for our realization and satisfaction. We forget that all of us have our common origin in divine existence and that we are mutually united on this plane. Instead of loving our fellow citizens, we begin to consider them as competitors or even enemies. Finally, we think that we have to protect ourselves, without letting certain people, situations or information come to us or enter us. We retract our receiving antennas so that we do not have to face challenges, and with this we cause a new contraction and the blocking of our chakras.

However, the need for recognition by our congeners or by a group to which we feel to belong is so intense that we are willing to guide our lives in broad areas according to the ideas of certain people close to us or according to generally accepted social rules, and to suppress our spontaneous feelings as soon as they cease to match expectations or conventions. This is only possible if we contract our chakras to such an extent that no controlled emotion can pass the filter. It then produces energy congestion in the affected chakra. Because energies can no longer radiate in their original form, they are distorted, break down the barrier and discharged inappropriately, in the form of intense and often negative emotions or an over-the-top activity boost.

This corresponds to a reaction to the blockage marked by the yang. But as if there is an expression of energies, into the chakra new energies can flow, which will be discharged in the same inappropriate way.

A reaction to the blockage of the chakras marked by the yin manifests itself in an almost absolute containment of energies, with which the energy flow practically paralyzes, since no space is created for the energies that flow later. The consequence is the undernourishment of vital energy and weakness in the manifestation of the affected chakra. The repercussions of similar hypofunction, as well as an overload of the corresponding chakras, can be found in the corresponding chapters of the chakras. There we will give some general guidelines that, in some points, may differ from your individual reactions, since they are ultimately determined by the experiences that have caused the blockage and that are stored in the emotional body and, in less measure, also in the mental body.

These stored experiences are not left behind by us with physical death. We drag them from one incarnation to the next, until we have polished them in the course of our evolution. They largely determine the circumstances in which we are reborn and the experiences we unconsciously attract in our new life through the irradiation of our emotional body.

However, in each life we have the possibility to dissolve very quickly, from childhood itself, our emotional structures. In a new-born, the entire energy system is still completely open and permeable. This means that in principle every born-again soul receives a new opportunity to lead a fulfilling life. But it also means that it is open to all vibrations and experiences, and with it also to all kinds of the imprint.

A new-born cannot yet consciously participate in the configuration of his life, nor can he relativize his experiences. Therefore, it is totally dependent on the goodwill and care of adults. Here lies for parents a great opportunity, and also a great task.

In the following pages we will describe what influences a child's needs in the first years of life to be able to develop optimally, to avoid new blockages and to dissolve old structures.

In our day, many highly evolved souls await suitable parents in which to incarnate without accumulating unnecessary blockages that could hinder the fulfillment of their mission on this earth. Other souls would like to be reincarnated in this time of ours of change, for they will hardly offer the self a similar opportunity to learn and grow again.

Knowing this can help prospective parents give a child-like soul the best starting possibilities for the way of life. But it can also help each of us better understand our own "history of blockages" and manage it more easily on this basis.

Already in the mother's womb, blockages in the energy system can begin when the incipient life is rejected, or when the mother lives in a permanent situation of stress, since a fetus lives and feels the world largely through the mother. A loving dedication to the little being found in the womb will provide your energy system with vibrations that will make you feel absolutely well and protected. When the mother lives the months of pregnancy happily, she is creating the optimal conditions for her child's life, in which she can fully discover her potential for happiness and creativity.

An important milestone in every person's life is the moment of birth. In certain circumstances, the experience of birth can mark us throughout a lifetime, and can be decisive for us to perceive the world as a friendly and pleasant place or as something hard, devoid of love and cold. With childbirth, the child abandons the complete physical security. During his first nine months of existence on earth, he has lived in a blissful state of timelessness and weightlessness, that provided him with food and protection. But the little being is ready for birth and curious about the world. Therefore, a natural birth, in which neither the mother nor the child is weakened by medicines, means great work and effort, but at the same time does not constitute a shock to the child. For which, however, it is not prepared at all for the separation of the mother immediately after birth. As long as the baby continues to feel the mother's body along with her familiar vibrations and sits cradled in the usual energetic vibrations of the mother's aura, she is ready to open herself with full confidence to new experiences.

In addition, body contact with the mother immediately after birth implies a deep bond between the mother and the child, which in specialized circles is called bonding. A flow of loving feelings, with positive emotional energy, flows automatically and without conscious participation from the mother to her new-born, and is not interrupted as long as the child feels the mother's body or stays at least within her emotional aura. This energy fills the little soul with confidence and joy. An interesting fact is that parents also develop more intimate contact with their babies and a more intuitive understanding when they have been present at birth and have been able to touch and caress the child.

Conversely, if the new-born is removed from the mother just after birth, he or she experiences deep pain from separation and loneliness. As long as the mother continues to consciously send her feelings and loving thoughts to the new-born during a separation, a contact will still be maintained, and the child will not be completely insulated from the mother's energetic supply. However, if she devotes her attention to other things or is tired or numb due to medications, this contact will also be broken.

The little creature senses its derelicts in an unknown and cold world in which it feels completely abandoned without the warm and protective presence of the mother. This experience is so violent that, in general, the child's energy system is not in a position to process terrible feelings, and experiences a profound impression, which results in the first blockage of energies. The blockage is preferably shown in the radical chakra area.

In the first year of life, when the child accumulates experiences predominantly through the physical body, the child needs first and foremost body contact with the mother, and sometimes also with the father or with other trusted people.

At this age the child does not yet have a concept of time. When she cries out of loneliness or hunger, she doesn't know if this state will end, and she easily despairs. On the other hand, if her demand is immediately met, the confidence that this earth provides children with everything they need to maintain their bodies and meet their physical needs is formed in her. The child can be opened, both physically and on the non-material plane, to the nourishing and protective energies available to us by our mother planet.

Practically, all primitive people have an intuitive knowledge of these relationships. They continually carry their babies wrapped in cloth by the body until they start crawling, and do not even abandon it when the continuous swinging has cradled and numbed the little creature. When the child starts crawling, they always lift him up as soon as the child wants it. At night the children stay with the mother in bed, and whenever they feel hungry, the mother's breast is at their service. The radiant eyes and satisfied faces of these happy little creatures speak for themselves. Children in these villages cry very rarely and are willing from an early age to take on social responsibility.

If in our society a mother also had this dedication during her child's first year of life and left her own needs in the background, she would have provided the creature with the best potential for her life. This investment is really worth it. The automatic flow of love and joy that is triggered in the mother through permanent body contact with the child is a broad compensation for all the little things he may not be able to do at that time.

If a child loses the original feelings of trust, safety, satisfaction, and protection, growing up, he will continue to look for them in the external and material realm. He will establish relationships with things rather than establishing them with people. It all starts with pets, which are used as a substitute for human closeness and heat. He then obtains more and more new toys and baubles, in an unconscious search for something to which he is driven by the slightly corrosive feeling of emptiness. And as adults, beautiful dresses, cars, furniture and perhaps a house of your own, as well as professional or social standing, are the things to which most men make their hearts more expensive, hoping to recover with them the feeling of security and abandoned childhood satisfaction. Our consumer society could not exist without that insatiable need for the vast majority of its members.

But the number of people who have realized that the experience of internal security and satisfaction cannot be achieved through material goods is also increasing. They set off for an inner quest, and here in fact lies the only chance to rediscover the lost paradise that most of us have abandoned with birth.

In the second year of life, the fundamental theme of the radical chakra, which extends over the first seven years of life, is joined by a new main theme of a single year. The growing child comes into contact with the energies of the second chakra. Delicate contact, caresses and pampering are now becoming more important, along with mere body contact. The child begins to discover his sensuality and to experience and express his sensations and emotions more consciously. From this moment the contents of the emotional body also begin to appear gradually, brought from the previous life. In his second year of life the child lives the most fundamental emotional structures in the first place.

It is now very important that parents do not try to impose a certain attitude on the child, because in that case he will start to retract emotions and suppress them in any way. If, on the other hand, the child learns to simply live his emotions, to accept the existence of them and to treat them playfully, he could dissolve in a short time all the negative emotional imprints.

Parents should understand that a child of that age does not express any negativity. If it gets choleric, it's only because a natural need has been disappointed. The raging cries and the legs release the blockage produced, and thus release the child. However, most parents find it difficult to accept their child as he is with his emotional expression, since they themselves do not have very clear things. They love their child when they do this or leave that, and with it they convey the following message: "Being like this you are not good enough."

The child assumes the attitude of the judgment of the parents, and because he does not want to lose his love, he relegates the parts of himself that are not dear. This results in a profound energy effect. If, in addition, sensory stimulation is lacking, a lack of original confidence arises in the emotional field and the sacral chakra is blocked.

Then the adult will find it difficult to accept and express his or her natural emotions. In order to feel something, you need a crude sensory stimulant, and you develop a tendency to observe others as objects that serve your own satisfaction.

The third year of life puts the little creature in contact with the energies of the solar plexus chakra. Emotional expression becomes more differentiated, and the explanations we have given regarding the second year of life only apply within certain limits. Now the child wants to prove himself as an independent personality, learns to know his influence and always says "no," to see what happens in that case.

When there is a power struggle between parents and the child because parents think that they can only educate the child by imposing their will on them, such a struggle culminates in the third year of life. If the child then does not feel loved and accepted in his growing personality, the energies of the solar plexus chakra are blocked. When you want to learn, you will lack the confidence and courage to live your individual personality, to configure your existence according to your own ideas and to learn from negative experiences. Instead, he will adapt or try to control his world.

Thus continues the journey of the little creature along with the energies of the different chakras. But let us leave these examples for now. With the help of the list of life cycles and with the description of each of the chakras, you will find it easy to complete the rest of the way yourself.

In all these explanations we should always bear in mind that it is us who have chosen the circumstances of our rebirth. We have embodied ourselves in a given couple to be properly polished, to gather experiences that our soul needs to develop towards perfection.

The fewer of us may have gone to parents who had such a deep understanding and a love so selfless that among their loving and expert hands, they melted, until the last restrictive structures of the emotional body disappeared. This means only the following: that in this life our mission and destiny are to develop the sympathetic love for ourselves that will dissolve the blockages and save the unwanted and imposed parts of our soul. Without being aware of this, our parents are the first teachers who, with their behavior, refer to our weaknesses, so that, based on pain and feelings of lack, we end up looking for ways to regain inner integrity. Then we take other people on this task and vital situations that we unconsciously attract, and that serves as a mirror for the anemic parts of us that we have repressed in the grim area of our psyche.

In the next chapter we will see the possibilities that exist to dissolve the chakra locks and rediscover the experience of inner unity.

CHAPTER 6

THE DISSOLUTION OF THE BLOCKAGES

There are essentially two ways to act on our chakras with a liberating and harmonizing effect. The first way is to expose the chakras to energetic vibrations that approach the frequencies with which a chakra naturally vibrates without blockages, and that works harmoniously. These energetic vibrations can be found, for example, in pure luminous colors, in precious stones, in sounds and essential oils, and also in the elements and multiple forms of manifestation of nature.

As soon as our chakras flow at frequencies that are higher and purer than those corresponding to their current state, they begin to vibrate more quickly, and the slower frequencies of the blockages gradually dissolve. Energy centers can absorb new vital energies and relay them unhindered to non-material bodies. It's as if, through our energy system, a cool breeze blows. The flowing prana charges the etheric body, which in turn transmits energy to the physical body. It also flows into the emotional body and the mental body, where blockages also begin to dissolve, as their vibrations are slower than those of the energy flowing into it. Finally, the pulse of vital energy affects the nadis of the entire energy system, and the body, spirit and soul begin to vibrate more highly, and radiate health and joy.

When stagnant energies are released in this process of purification and clarification, their contents appear once again in our consciousness. With this we can again live the same sensations that caused the blockage: our anxieties, our anger and our pain. Body diseases may come out for the last time before being completely cleaned. During these processes we probably feel uneasy, excited or even very tired. As soon as the energies have an expeditious way, they return to us deep joy, serenity and clarity.

However, many people do not have the courage to go through the necessary clarification processes. Often, they simply have no knowledge of them, and the experiences presented interpret them as a step backward in their evolution.

In fact, the blockages of our energy system are purified only to the extent that, since our complete evolution, we are willing to look to the face of the unwanted and repressed part of ourselves, and to redeem it through our love. And with this we come to the second way, which we mentioned at the beginning of this chapter. This route should permanently accompany the first path of direct activation and purification of chakras, but at the same time it is itself an independent possibility to harmonize our internal energy system and free it from blockages.

This path is the inner attitude of unconditional acceptance, which leads to complete détente. Tension implies the opposite, the remedy against tension, against contraction, and against blocking. As long as we consciously or unconsciously reject any scope of ourselves, as long as we prosecute ourselves, and therefore count and reject parts of ourselves, a tension will remain that prevents complete bloating and, therefore, both, the dissolution of the blockages.

We've all met more than once with people who say they can't relax. These people permanently need distraction or activity, even in their free time or on vacation, and when they ever do nothing there is always inner dialogue. As soon as they reach peace externally they feel an inner unease. In these people the self-healing mechanism is so active that the blockages begin to dissolve immediately as soon as some peace of mind is established in the energy system. However, because the people affected do not understand this mechanism, they flee again and again to the activity, thus suppressing the processing and purification of blocked energies.

Other people encapsulate their mental bodies to circumvent confrontation with the contents of their emotional body. For these people, all experiences take place through understanding. They analyze, interpret and categorize, but never get into an experience with their whole being.

We also sometimes encounter people who have tried to force the opening of the chakras by practicing disproportionately and without being guided by anyone. For example, certain exercises of Kundalini yoga, and they end up flooded with the contents unconscious of the corresponding chakra. Attempts to reject these contents can sometimes lead to deeper blockages. It is also not uncommon for someone who has started a spiritual path to only activate their upper chakras and unconsciously maintain the blockages of the lower chakras, since they do not want to identify with the contents that are released. One of these may have access to wonderful experiences from the realms of his upper chakras, and yet he may feel deep inside him a lack or void. Unconditional joy, the feeling of complete life joy and safety in life can only arise if all chakras are uniformly open and their frequencies vibrate on the highest possible plane.

However, the attitude of unconditional acceptance demands a great deal of honesty and courage. Honesty means in this context the willingness to see ourselves with all our weaknesses and negativity, and not as we would like to see ourselves. Value is the willingness to accept the observed. It's the value of saying yes to everything without excluding anything.

We have assumed in us the judgments of our parents to win their love. We have suppressed certain emotions and desires of ours to meet the expectations of society, a group or an image of ourselves. Abandoning this means orienting ourselves inwardly and absolutely, and losing the love and recognition of others. But it is only the act of rejection, of denial, that allows our energies to adopt negative manifestations. Repressed emotions only become "bad" because we reject them, rather than face them with love and understanding. The more violently they are rejected, both "worse" and mortifying will they be, until at some point we release them from prison through our love.

Behind all sentimental stimulus is, ultimately, the drive to regain the original paradisiac state of unity. However, as soon as we adapt to the prevailing worldview and only accept as real the external plane of reality that can be perceived through our physical senses and rational understanding, this desire for communion, of unification with life, becomes a will to possess. Our eagerness to possess a person, a position, love and recognition and material goods, however, is disappointed again and again, or in the long run is not satisfied as expected, since such satisfaction can only be achieved through an inner union.

For fear of a new disappointment we suppress our energies: our energy system is blocked. The energies that subsequently flow are distorted by the blockage and manifest themselves as negative emotions, which in turn we try, once again, to repress and retain so as not to lose the sympathy of our fellow citizens.

We can interrupt this circle if we devote all our attention to our emotions. At that very moment they begin to transform, for finally, we recognize that they are simply energies that have arisen from the desire for unity, and that were blocked in their original manifestation. Now they become a force that helps us continue on the path to totality.

There is a simple analogy that can clarify these relationships. If you're afraid of a person and you shun them, you'll never know them in their entire being. If, on the other hand, you devote your attention to them and make them feel your unconditional love, they will open to you gradually. You will know that after their negative behaviours, which you have condemned, there is nothing but the longing for disappointed satisfaction. Your understanding will help you walk the path to real satisfaction. In this analogy, your emotions happen the same as that person.

The written attitude of acceptance without prejudice corresponds to the position of our higher self. As we consciously assume it for ourselves, we open ourselves to the vibration plane of the inner guidance in us and entrust it with the mission of guiding us to a whole and healthy existence.

The higher self is that part of the soul that binds us to divine existence. It's unlimited in space and time. For this reason, it has access at all times to the integral knowledge that affects both life in the universe and our personal life. If we entrust ourselves to our guide, it will lead us to the straightest and most direct way towards the inner unit, and the existing blockages in our energy system will dissolve as smoothly as possible.

If we understand these relationships, we can make the forms of therapy described in this book effective. Always admit all the experiences that appear during the performance of therapy, even (and more if possible) when they appear at an unpleasant or negative time; give them your neutral attention and your love and give them the healing power of your higher self.

There are forms of meditation that can help you practice this attitude of acceptance, dissolve blockages, and admit the self-healing energies of your higher self. One of these meditation techniques, is transcendental meditation, also known by its abbreviation, MT. Here, consciousness is guided without any effort or concentration of any kind by the most direct way towards the experience of the pure being. This process is accompanied by a growing relaxation in which the blocked energies dissolve on their own. The liberated thoughts and emotions are not rejected, but are continually replaced by the experience of increasing relaxation and joy. With this meditation, you have in your hands a wonderful and highly effective instrument that, used correctly, represents by itself a way to activate your chakras harmoniously, to purify your energy system from all blockage and to explore all your intellectual and mood potential. However, this form of meditation can only be learned through a qualified teacher.

There are also other forms of meditation that can help you on your way. Keep in mind that in the meditation you choose, your thoughts and feelings are not prosecuted and rejected, but integrated as part of the necessary cleansing process. Even in the most effective and natural forms of meditation, it can happen that, due to habit, there is always some judgment. Even experiences resulting from the dissolution of blockages can often be unconsciously suppressed, as they have felt unpleasant. This can cause you to lose impartiality, and the effectiveness of meditation will suffer. An experienced teacher can help you find the original meditation experience again.

As soon as you have learned to love and accept yourself entirely, as you are, you will radiate these vibrations through your aura, and attract the corresponding experiences in the outside world. This means that only then will you really gain the love and recognition of others, whose loss you may have feared before. They begin to value you as you are in your true essence, and admire you for your true value of being yourself. Authentic love and communion are only possible under this premise.

Here's one last point in relation to the subject of this chapter. On your way to an integral evolution, there can be phases in which your chakras are relatively open without all the blockages being dissolved. So you are very sensitive to the energies that fall within the scope of your aura, but you still do not radiate enough luminous energy to attract only profitable energies to be able to neutralize negative energies in your environment.

If you remain now in a tense atmosphere where vibrations of dissatisfaction, hostility or aggressiveness prevail, your chakras can be loaded with negative energies, or contracted to protect themselves from such influxes. In both cases, the consequence is a positive vital energy underfeeding.

As soon as the energy fields of two people touch or overlap, there is an immediate exchange and mutual influence of energies. We unconsciously perceive the other energetically, whether we want to or not. When a person is spontaneously sympathetic or unfriendly to us, it is largely due to the energetic vibrations we experience in their aura. If we feel fear, dissatisfaction or anger, these vibrations not only influence the image we have of it, but also our own energy system. When, for no apparent reason, you feel tense or uncomfortable in the presence of a person; and you even get the feeling that everything contracts within you, the reason is in the irradiation of your aura. If, on the contrary, in a person's aura you feel joy, love and serenity, in their presence you will feel particularly well, even if you do not exchange any words with them. In a group of people who have gathered for a particular purpose, the collective aura that arises can have such an intense effect that all the members of the group are reached by it. Suffice it to think of the contagious environment that occurs so often among the viewers of a football match.

On the other hand, when a group meets for devotion or common meditation, the individual can rise to planes of consciousness far higher than those corresponding to their normal state of evolution.

Places also have their own irradiation, since matter can store vibrations. This happens especially in enclosed spaces.

We believe that when dealing with young children it is particularly important to understand these relationships. The energy system of these small beings is not yet completely sensitive to all kinds of energy vibrations. It reacts in a particularly sensitive way to every loving thought and to any feeling of joy, but also to aggressions or quarrels and to the aggressiveness of its environment. Here the body closeness to a parent or a reference person with whom you are familiar represents valuable protection: for example, when the child is exposed to vibrations of others when going shopping. The adult's aura acts as a bumper that captures and absorbs vibrations. For this reason, it is better to carry a child than to leave him/her in a baby stroller.

We adults can also contribute a lot to making our own chakras and our children's chakras remain relaxed and open. When we fundamentally attract those vibrations and situations that correspond to our own energy radiation, we also have a certain space of action to consciously shape our life in the exterior aspect. For example, we can participate in activities in which an atmosphere of joy and love is generated, we can visit places that radiate positive and uplifting energy, and we can even create the enchantment of a similar place in our own home. Stimulating colors, flowers, aromas and soothing music contribute a lot to a harmonious and flattering atmosphere of life. By choosing the TV shows, conversations and activities we develop within our four walls, we can put certain accents and create an atmosphere in which the energy system of all the people present recovers from negative influences.

Also, internally, you can do something to protect yourself especially from unwanted influencers from the environment. We recommend that you pay special attention to therapy to open the heart chakra, since the love that radiates outward is able to neutralize or transform all negative vibrations. Here is a special challenge to develop your love together with other faculties.

In addition, when you develop your heart chakra, you will know and evaluate more and more the positive sides of other people, and you will automatically let into you only those vibrations. Through your assessment, these qualities will be enhanced and activated at the same time on your opponent. Thus, each encounter can become an enrichment for both parties.

Active outward irradiation in all cases represents good protection. As soon as you have learned to accept yourself as you are and openly radiate your energies, the external negative vibrations will not be able to penetrate the crown of lightning that emerged from you. If you remain inwardly relaxed and completely calm, the tensions of the atmosphere will not find any echo essential in you and will not be able to settle inside you or influence you negatively.

Of course, we are aware that these capabilities presuppose a truly advanced evolution. That's why we want to mention some more simple possibilities with which you can protect yourself from unwanted influences and keep negative energies away.

When you want to protect yourself in a situation or intensify your own influence, imagine that you introduce light into your body through your coronal chakra, and let that light radiate from your solar plexus chakra again, wrapping your body in a controller luminous protector that will dissolve all dark influences. You can also imagine the luminous radiation coming from the solar plexus chakra as if it were a shower or a spotlight or a projector that eliminates all negative vibrations in its path.

Another very effective protection is that offered by essential oils; you should apply these directly to the chakras. They fill your aura with pure irradiation and neutralize un-harmonic tensions and influences, from the outside to your aura.

Carrying a rock crystal with you will enhance the luminous quality and protective irradiation force of your aura. Its effect complements very well with the influence of essential oils.

Silk underwear is also energy protection, and is especially recommended for infants and young children. If you ever get too tight due to a sudden scare, shock or anger, here's a very effective

CHAKRAS HEALING FOR BEGINNERS

possibility that will allow you to immediately eliminate stagnant energies. Sit with your legs slightly outstretched and for a few seconds tighten as many muscles as possible. If you're alone, shout as loud as you want; otherwise, just expel air from your lungs with intense pressure. Repeat this exercise until you feel better. It serves to dissolve the blockages that have arisen because your energy system could not process the sudden experience. If you've done well, then you can stretch hard, as you do after a deep, restful sleep. It is interesting that in some people the phenomenon of muscle tension appears spontaneously in meditation, and precisely in those regions of the body where blockages want to be dissolved. This is a clear sign of the usefulness and effectiveness of this exercise.

CHAPTER 7

HOW WE CAN DETECT THE CHAKRAS WE HAVE BLOCKED

As in this book, we offer several possibilities to harmonize and balance your chakras, of course, it is of great interest to know if your chakras are unbalanced or blocked, and which of them are. If you don't know, you could harmonize all the chakras with the possible therapies on offer, and we highly recommend this method of comprehensive treatment. But if, for example, you have detected that there are two chakras that prefer to need therapy, you can dedicate yourself predominantly to those two energy centers.

In addition, the knowledge of dissonant chakras hides a great opportunity for self-knowledge, which can be fully opened to those who are interested. This is always, first, about ourselves, and only secondly to others, to whom, of course, we can tell our experiences. However, the goal is not to convert others, but to know and save oneself, and then to be able to lovingly lead others on the same path of self-knowledge.

For the diagnosis of chakras, we are offered several different possibilities. So using one of those opportunities will be enough to perform a self-diagnosis or effective diagnosis of the chakra system.

1) In this book, when describing each of the chakras, we give clear characteristics for recognition, in which you can measure which of your chakras are dissonant, harmonized or functioning defectively. With the help of these criteria, anyone can know their problem areas quickly. We have tried very clearly, sometimes even in an exaggerated way, to outline the repercussions of a dysfunction of the chakras, to clarify certain trends quickly and unequivocally. When reading further, you should also consider that not all the repercussions described apply to anyone. However, it may happen that you feel very affected by certain passages of text or feel that they don't affect you at all. That's not our goal. However, we want to get you to recognize yourself clearly and unequivocally, and that when some of the descriptions are correct in your particular case, they make you feel involved. Please do not value this as a reproach of ours directed against you, for the goal is not to hurt you, but to help you gain knowledge. However, self-knowledge is not always pleasant; also, sometimes our gloomy sides must be illuminated, for only in this way can they be released. So this way for

knowledge will be worth it, without a doubt, since at the same time it puts in your hands a whole series of possibilities for the self-treatment of chakras and the self-harmonization of them.

2) Another possibility to analyze our chakra system is to carefully observe which chakras react strikingly in situations of extraordinary stress or shock. It could be that, in certain difficult life situations, you will always be assaulted by the same ailments: for example, if the radical chakra is hyperfunctioning, in a strong situation of effort you can have the feeling of "losing foot," which may even give you diarrhea. In the case of hyperfunction of the first chakra, it is easy to be assaulted by anger and aggressive outbursts. If in your second chakra there is a lack of functioning, in the face of extraordinary tensions there is a blockage of feelings; with an exaggerated function, you will in all likelihood break down in tears or react with uncontrolled emotionality. In the case of hypofunction in the third chakra, in the face of great efforts, a feeling of impotence, a feeling of incapacity, or an uncomfortable sensation in the stomach or a stubborn nervousness will be established. An overload in this chakra is characterized by nerve excitability and the attempt to control the situation through hyperactivity. If you get the feeling that "your heart stops," you have to blame it on a hypofunction of the coronal chakra.

When your heart is broken in the face of stress, it's an indication of a generalized dysfunction of the fourth chakra. In the case of hypofunction of the neck chakra, you get a lump in your throat, you will probably start to stutter or your head will shake uncontrollably; in the event of dissonant hyperfunction, you will try to take the situation firmly by means of an avalanche of unripe words. If in situations of stress or shock you cannot have clear ideas, it means a hypofunction of the frontal chakra and an overload would often be expressed with headaches.

Such reactions always occur only in the weaknesses of our energy system. An interesting observation can open our eyes to these cases.

3) Now we can continue to use body language. For the first time it is possible to determine, by the external form and by the external qualities of a person's body, whether any area is energetically in dissonance. At the end of the day, our body is a perfect mirror image of non-material energy structures. Whenever bodily abnormalities occur, whether spasms, swellings, tensions, weaknesses or the like, we can assign them to the corresponding chakra depending on where they occur. We all know the differences in bodily appearances that we can use to form a clear image of

the particular person; often, spontaneously and without reflection. Frequently, this image can be easily transferred to the chakras. Thus, we find people who obviously have all their energy oriented upwards, and who in the lower part of the body have absolutely weak characteristics. In others, the exact opposite is true; and there are also others that seem to be composed only of weaknesses or strengths. Observe yourself sometimes, consciously, in the mirror or in photographs. Voice is often an important criterion for prosecuting the state of the neck chakra.

If you also take into account the organic weaknesses or even the symptoms of the disease, you have one of the most transparent reference points on what is the area of the chakra system where deficiencies exist, to effectively apply the therapy.

4) As a fourth possibility, we put in your hand a special test with which many therapists work, in addition to a large number of laypeople. For this, you usually need two people, placed face to face. This is a kinesiological test, which was developed in the course of the Touch for Health method.

In practice, it proceeds as follows: place your right hand on a chakra and simultaneously laterally extend the left arm to the right angle with the body. The other person doing the test with you gives the order to "oppose resistance," and while you try to keep your arm in the right position, she tries to push her arm down, exerting pressure at about wrist height. If the chakra is harmonized and balanced in its operation, the extended arm offers a clear and intense resistance; if, on the other hand, the chakra being tested is blocked, it can be easily noticed that the arm does not oppose this resistance, and the person performing the test will be able to push it down with very little force.

Kinesiological Muscle Test

Through this test method we can go through the seven chakras, from the radical chakra to the coronal chakra; which allows us to get a clear picture of the energetic state of the chakras. When there are disorders in the chakra, in the test, the arm always reacts with weakness. We can then repeat this same test to find that there are changes. With a disorders chakra system, the arm test should give the "strong" result seven times: that is, the down pushed arm should offer sensitive resistance seven times. You can pause briefly between tests of the different chakras to prevent possible phenomena of arm fatigue.

Measurements made with a special kinesiometer have shown the result that a similar test resists approximately 20-kilogram pressure, if the test result is 'strong'; Otherwise, the arm will no longer offer resistance with approximately 8 kilograms of pressure. Of course, account must be taken of the individual physical constitution of the person subject to the test. However, the difference between 'strong' and 'weak' will be clearly perceived both by the person undergoing the test and by the person administering the test.

Another variant of this test is to hold down the thumb against the index finger of the right hand, and with the left hand cover the chakra object of the test. Our companion in the test will try, when the relevant order is given, to separate the fingers that we hold firmly tight against each other. If the fingers offer great resistance, the chakra under test is in good condition. If, on the contrary, the resistance is reduced, the chakra tested is disrupted and needs therapy.

However, we have often found people who perform this test with themselves. To do this they press the index finger against the thumb of one hand, and try to separate them with the thumb and index finger of the other. In doing so they are mentally concentrated in a given chakra. Also here it is clearly shown by the feeling of "weakness" or "strength," which chakra is deranged. If the fingers that are pressed against each other can be released by the other hand ("weak"), the chakra being tested is deranged. If the fingers remain firmly united ("strong"), the chakra is in good condition. It is true that for these kinesiological tests we need some practice if we are to achieve safe results. However, this method works excellently, and serves to recognize well in which of the chakras we should work to harmonize it.

5) We will call "internal vision" another possibility that we have to prosecute our chakras. For many people it is the easiest and fastest way to get in touch with your energy system.

To do this, we go into a meditative state of silence for a few minutes and try to form an idea of the state of each of the chakras through our "inner eyes." In doing so, we systematically and slowly traverse the chakras, from the bottom to the top. Many people can clearly recognize the status of their chakras based on chromatic changes. Other people tend to see shapes. If this is your case, look at whether they are round and have a harmonic balance, or if they have intussusceptions or show other variations. And, in turn, there are other people who recognize the harmonic state of the chakras by their size and power of irradiation. A combination of these different elements is often perceived. All these possibilities and valuation criteria are, however, based on a certain self-experience, and need to be trained often, if we want to come up with unequivocal and clear results.

6) More and more people are able to feel with their hands the energetic situation of the chakras. It feels a certain resistance when it is impacted with the energy envelope of your own etheric body, in which the chakras settle, or with the energy envelope of another person. This resistance feels similar to what happens when moving in water. You may be able to detect certain roughness, holes, or excrement. We can practice it by slowly bringing hands closer to our own body, to another person's body or even to animals and plants, and trying to sensory-perceive the changes that are being operated on. Also, in this case, the experience born of the frequent application of the technique itself is essential for clear divination. A workshop in this regard would be advisable.

7) The most direct path we may well consider to be 'providence,' even if only a relatively small number of people possess this gift. Through this power the "seer" has direct access to the energy situations and processes that are consumed in himself and in other people. It is possible to know and value both the bodily references and the intellectual ones. If you

count on the blessing of these media faculties, it is of great importance to interpret correctly what is observed and for this it takes a lot of training, experience and a gift of observation.

If you are not completely sure whether or not you have these faculties, you can do the following tests: sit in a completely dark room, for example, in a basement, a sauna or even a scot-in closet, where the slightest light does not penetrate. Stay in it silently for several minutes. As objects for testing, some rock crystal tips placed at a certain distance or held in the hands are sufficient at first. If you are able to perceive certain subtle energy radiations at the tips of rock crystals, especially when moving with swing motion, it is indicative of a tendency to clairvoyance. Don't give in to the first, because sometimes this ability has to be trained. First of all, this exercise should be done completely stress-free. If you want to detect the energetic body around a person, a predominantly black background should be preferred, to which the person being tested sits or stands. From a few meters away, looking in the direction of the person, or better through it, since that is where the energetic crown, the aura, is located. The best results will be obtained in a certain meditative state.

Take your time for it. Presumably, in this exercise you

will first detect the etheric body, which envelops the physical body as a radiant energy envelope. With some practice you will also be able to distinguish the colors and shapes of the emotional body. Don't expect any fixed or rigid color image, since non-material energies are in continuous motion and have predominantly translucent intense gloss qualities. Basically, it can be said that the harmonic colors and shapes in this energetic image allow the existence of a harmonious person to be concluded; unsharp colors and undefined shapes point to that person's problematic areas.

If you want to try to detect your own aura, you can stand in front of a wall mirror and carry out the corresponding studies. Most people find it easier to achieve this by first looking at someone else's energy radiation.

In addition, there are special glasses for auras, which have dark violet glasses with a wrap that makes them airtight and opaque around. These glasses should be classified as auxiliary means; they don't automatically open access to non-material plans to all users, but they can really help us move up to them.

More and more people are in a position to judge and evaluate the energetic body, and in particular the system of other people's chakras, even at great distances, several hundred or even thousands of kilometers. In general, this is done through a photo of the consultant, or also through the phone.

If it causes you trouble recognizing or understanding such extraordinary phenomena, think about all that is possible today, for example, thanks to radio and television. Also, here, images and sounds are sent and captured invisibly through the ether in the form of waves. Almost all of our technical developments previously existed as natural phenomena, as did wireless transmission.

And, of course, it is up to your free will to reject the methods and possibilities that you find difficult for you, since a whole series of different possibilities of analysis referring to chakras have previously been shown.

8) Another way to detect the functioning of someone else's chakras is the medial ability to perceive in our own chakras exactly what our consultant experiences and feels. To do this, the therapist first goes into resonance with the patient's energetic body. There are some therapists who work like this and make clear diagnoses. However, not a few of them feel bad after the appointment, suffering the same symptom as the consultant. Hence, preference should be given to other procedures.

9) Some traditional Asian texts mention different characteristics of a dominant foundation of specific chakras. In this regard it is particularly interesting to analyze our sleep habits.

When a person lives, above all, through his first chakra, in general he will have quite large sleep needs, ranging from 10 to 12 hours, and will prefer to sleep upside down. People who need approximately 8 to 10 hours of sleep, and preferably sleep in the fetal position, live predominantly through the second chakra. When life is first and foremost configured by the third chakra, they preferably sleep on their back, and natural sleep needs range from 7 to 8 hours. A man whose fourth chakra is widely developed usually lies on the left side, and needs approximately 5 or 6 hours of sleep per night. If the fifth chakra is open and it is the one that sets the pattern, he only falls asleep 4 to 5 hours per night, alternating between the right or left side position. When in a person the sixth chakra is open, active and dominant, he will only spend approximately 4 hours between sleep and wakefulness. Watchful sleep is a state in which inner consciousness is maintained while the body sleeps. This form of rest is what you would expect with a seventh open and dominant chakra. The fully enlightened, therefore, does not sleep in the usual sense of the term; in any case, if you give your body a resting phase.

So, through these features, we are able to check the functioning of our chakras.

Alongside the possibilities shown there are some other technical means of support from the para scientific sector. These include the pendulum and magic wand, as well as The Kirlian photograph, which some therapists resort to performing the analysis of the chakras. Among the magic wands, one of the most suitable is the so-called zahorí pendulum, which is also called a biosensor. With this device, the state of the chakras can be known with relative ease, as with a pendulum: a stable chakra will manifest itself by the large circles it produces in the pendulum or wand, and an altered chakra, by minor circles or even because the pendulum or wand are rested. Of course, here it is also necessary to practice a little to be able to clearly differentiate the results.

Kirlian photography is a special technical procedure that allows us to obtain photographs of energy radiation, for example, of our body, and to represent them in colors. Recently a really interesting diagnostic possibility has been developed from this method. The diagnosis of energy terminal points by healer, Peter Mandel, is currently of great interest. Meanwhile, a large number of doctors and healers already work through this bioenergy diagnostic method.

Sophisticated electronic systems are already being used in Japan to arrive at the corresponding diagnostics in the field of non-material. But since we are more confident in our own interior possibilities, we only mention in passing these technical auxiliary means.

At the end of the day, so that only one of the methods presented here to check the chakras will be useful to you, it can be more than enough. It is often better to properly master one thing than several half-hearted things. So we wish you to be able to apply this knowledge sensibly.

CHAPTER 8

SEXUALITY AND CHAKRAS

Human sexuality is a form of manifestation and a mirror of the perpetual act of creation that is consumed uninterruptedly on all the planes of the da in the universe. When at the moment of creation multiplicity emerged from unity, the amorphous being was first divided into two fundamental forms of energy: a male fertilizer and a spawning female force. A few thousand years ago, the Chinese gave these original forces the denomination of yin and yang. From the game of these energies comes creation. The female yin is continuously fertilized by the male seed of yang and engenders life in its infinitely varied forms.

On a physical level of man, this game of forces manifests itself as sexuality. Through it, man is united in its entirety with the perpetual act of creating life, and the ecstasy he can experience in it reflects the blessing of creation.

The forces of yin and yang manifest the most universe as polarity. In order to exist, everything has an opposite pole. Each of the poles exists only by the other pole; if one polarity disappears, so does the other. This fundamental rule can apply to everything. For example, we can only breathe out if we also breathe in; if we leave one of them, we are also deprived of the other; the interior conditions the outside; day conditions the night; light conditions the shadow; birth, death; women, men, etc., with both polarities being mutually interchangeable. Each pole needs to be complemented by the opposite.

Yin and yang very intuitively symbolize the rhythmic movement of a lifetime. The yin represents the face of the whole, the feminine, extensive, intuitive, passive and unconscious; the yang represents the male, concentrator, intellectual, active and conscious. However, no assessment is included here in the sense of 'having more value than the other.'

The balance that exists in the universe around us is the result of the relationships between opposing couples. As in this universe everything is in a perpetual flow of motion, both yin and yang are already present latently at the corresponding opposite pole. This is symbolized by the white dot inside the dark yin, and by the dark point inside the white yang. Each of the two poles conceals the opposite pole in the form of seed, and it is only a matter of time when one of the polarities will be transformed into the corresponding other. In some areas, this investment is consumed in fractions of a second, such as at the atomic level. In humans, this change of polarity, from male to female, or vice versa, is only possible through various incarnations. Day and night need on average twelve hours to make such a change, and inspiration and exhalation only a few seconds.

Reversing polarities

All things come and go, as well as move and change due to the exchange and interaction of these two fundamental forces of the universe. But only both cycles result in the entire unit.

Love and sexuality are also founded by this regular law. Two poles merge into the unit, attracting each other like the different poles of a magnet. If a union of the opposing forces occurs, they are exchanged with each other. Women and men have opposite polarization in all their fundamental features. This different polarization also exists on the energy plane. Wherever the man presents a positive pole, the woman is endowed with a negative pole, and vice versa. As already explained in the introductory chapter, this phenomenon also occurs in the direction of rotation of chakras (in homosexuality, for example, there is an energy polarization opposite to the norm).

91

Thus, between the woman and the man there is an attraction and complementation in all the planes represented by the chakras, which can lead to complete intimate fusion. To achieve it, however, chakras must be as free from blockages as possible. In sexual union, the energetic flow along the main channel, Sushumna, is strongly aroused and intensified. The energy flow of the second chakra increases greatly and, when there are no blockages in the chakra system, it is energy-intensive and loads all other chakras. Here sexual energy, which represents a certain form of prana, is transformed into the frequencies of the remaining chakras. From the chakras, and through the nadis, it radiates in the physical body and towards the energetic body, and fills them with multiplied life force. At the climax of this union there is a violent mutual discharge of energy through the seven chakras and fusion in all planes, represented by the chakras. Both partners feel enlivened to the depths of their being and at the same time totally relaxed; they feel an intimate union and a love that goes beyond the personal will to possess. The relationship is consummated without relying on the external things.

Such a satisfactory sexual union can only be lived in this dimension when the partners give each other completely and free the self from any anguish that could hinder the free flow in the energy system. It is sufficient that a single chakra is blocked in one of the components of the couple so that the union cannot be experienced in all its completeness. The blocked chakra also causes an alteration of the energy flow of the same chakra in the companion.

Most people only live sexuality through the second chakra. In man, too, the energy of the radical chakra plays a dominant role as a physical instinctive force. However, if sexuality is limited to the lower chakra, it becomes a rather one-sided experience, from which both companions are basically weakened and dissatisfied, and have a tendency to quickly separate and continue on their own. It's as if, on a string instrument, only two strings are crossed, but the full range of sounds was never taken out. From an energetic point of view, in limited sexual practice, in this way a lot of energy is actually consumed, since energies are extracted from other chakras and transformed into sexual energy, and then irradiated through the second chakra. The energies are unable to take their natural path upwards and simultaneously enter the seven chakras to fill them with additional vital energy.

The most natural way to dissolve the blockages that prevent a perfect sexual union in all planes is an exchange of energies of the heart chakra. When both partners radiate the love of their hearts freely and without fear, their own energy system, just like the other person's, is harmonized in the eyes of their own energy system. Blockages caused by distress dissolve, and it is possible to exchange the planes of the seven chakras.

Here's the deeper reason why the sexual union is experienced as very satisfying when, in addition to physical attraction, there is a feeling of deep love between the couple's partners. The higher frequencies are activated and sexuality rises beyond being purely bodily together, to become a spiritual union.

This is the art of tantra, taught and practiced for millennia. Here we come to a wide-ranging violent orgasmic experience that is generally considered possible. Such an experience actually leads us to areas of another dimension of experience and feeling. Suddenly we are aware that sexual energies are not enclosed in our genitals. They exist in each of our cells, just as the game of female and male forces exists in all forms of manifestation of creation. The perfect union with a beloved partner leads us to the experience of inner uniqueness with the life that throbs in the universe. And in the instant of orgasm, when duality is suppressed for a moment, we live in unity with the absolute and amorphous being, which constitutes the permanent basis and the goal of polarities.

The first chakra and its correspondences

Keywords: Physical energy and will to live. Survival instinct. Fight, strength, stability, integration. Setting goals on Earth. To be and to have. Be. Material consciousness, the limitation for manifestation, discipline. Development and nutrition. Rest and food. Simple physical comfort, pleasure, and health.

- Location: In the perineum, between the anus and the genitals.
- Sanskrit name: Muladhara.
- Sound: lam.
- Phoneme: o
- Verb: I have.
- Colors: Blood red activates it, green calms it.
- Foods: Proteins in general (meat, lentils, soy).
- Essential oils: Patchouli, cedar, cloves.

- Gems: All red (garnet, red jasper, obsidian, smoky quartz).
- Corresponding element: Earth
- Sensory function: Smell
- Symbol: Four-petal loto
- Basic principle: Bodily will for being (as a polar opposite to the spiritual will to be in the seventh chakra).
- Body correspondences: All solid, such as the spine, bones, teeth and nails; and, rectum, large intestine, prostate, blood and cell structure.
- Corresponding glands: Adrenal glands

The adrenal glands produce adrenaline and norepinephrine, which have the mission of adapting blood circulation to specific needs by regulating blood distribution. In this way the body is prepared for action and can react immediately to the demands posed. In addition, the adrenal glands have a predominant influence on the body's thermal balance.

Astrological correspondences:

- Aries/Mars: Reboot, original vital energy, force to impose, aggression.
- Taurus: Linkage with the earth, possession, sensory enjoyment.

- Scorpio/Pluto: Unconscious link, sexual strength, transformation and renewal.
- Capricorn/Saturn: Structure, resistance.

In Ayurveda, the radical chakra is also assigned to the Sun, as the original giver of life.

Mission and operation of the first chakra

The radical chakra binds us to the physical world. It directs cosmic energies on the earthly corporeal plane, while simultaneously the earth's energy flows through it into the non-material energy system.

Here we come into contact with the spirit of "Mother Earth," we experience her elemental strength, her love and her patience.

The fundamental needs of life and survival, both individual and global, on this planet fall within the scope of action of the first chakra.

The "if" to life on earth, to physical existence, and the willingness to act in harmony with the energy of the Earth and learn from it are gifts of a first open chakra.

Thus the radical chakra is assigned to the earth element, its color is the red of energy and activity, of the most intimate nucleus of our planet. It gives us earthly security and the "safe ground" under our feet, on which we can build our lives, and simultaneously provides us with the energy necessary for creative activity in the world. It also gives us the strength to impose ourselves and perseverance.

The construction of existence, material assurance and the "preservation of one's own species" through the foundation of a family also fall within the scope of action of the first chakra, as well as sexuality as a bodily function and as a means for Procreation.

The radical chakra forms the most important foundation of life and the source of vital energy for the upper chakras. Here we are united with the inexhaustible energy reserve of Kundalini energy. It also starts the three main channels, Sushumna, Ida and Pingala. Like our heart in the physical body, the basal chakra is the central point of our non-material energy circulation system. In addition, it is where the collective subconscious settles, to which memorized knowledge we have access to here. It should be compensated with the seventh chakra, to maintain the inner balance of man.

Harmonic operation

When your radical chakra is open and functioning harmoniously, you experience a deep and personal union with the Earth and its creatures, an unclouded life force, a being based on yourself and life, satisfaction, stability and inner strength. You feel immersed in the natural cycle of life, in the alternation of rest and activity, of death and of the new birth. Your actions are carried out by the desire to participate creatively in the configuration of life on your mother planet, in line with the generating power of the earth, with life in nature. It's easy for you to accomplish your goals in the world. Your life is driven by an imperturbable original trust. You live on the earth as a safe place where you receive everything you need: dedication, food, safety and protection. Thus you open yourself with confidence to life on this earth and accept gratefully all that she has in her right standing for you.

When there is a unilateral accentuation or dysfunction of the radical chakra, your thinking and action revolve predominantly around material possession and safety, as well as around sensory stimuli and pleasures, such as: good food, alcoholic beverages, sex, etc. Everything you long for, you would want to acquire without thinking about the consequences. At the same time, you may find it difficult to give and receive frankly. You have a tendency to protect yourself and delimit yourself. Not infrequently the non-detachable and the desire to retain manifests itself on the body plane in the form of constipation and overweight.

Your action is predominantly aimed at satisfying only your own needs. And you ignore, or unconsciously overlook, the needs of others and your own body for a healthier and more moderate diet, sufficient rest, and a balanced, harmonious way of life.

In the extreme case, you cling to certain ideas and ambitions from which you cannot part. When your bindings are challenged by circumstances or others, you react by easily extolling and getting angry. And in extreme situations, also in an angry and aggressive way. The violent imposition of one's own desires and ideas also falls within the scope of a deranged radical chakra.

Anger and violence are ultimately defense mechanisms that point to an original lack of trust. Behind it is always the anguish of losing something or even not receiving something, which transmits security and well-being.

The Earth is, for you, a place that must be dominated and exploited, to ensure the survival of man. Thus, the prey that is exercised today with the forces of the Earth, and the destruction of its natural balance, are symptoms of a radical chakra alteration in most modern men.

Hypofunction

With a locked or closed radical chakra, your body build is quite weak and you have little physical and mood resistance. A lot of things in life worry you, and you know the feelings of insecurity all too well. You may also have the feeling of not stepping on dry land, you feel "elevated" or "not present." It's not easy for you to deal with life's challenges, and you often lack the capacity to impose yourself as well as stability. So often life on this earth seems to you as a burden and not a joy. You almost always yearn for a life that is easier, more enjoyable and less demanding.

In case you have unilaterally developed your upper chakras, a hypofunction of the radical chakra can convey the feeling of not belonging very well to this Earth. Since you can only hardly capture the earth's elemental vital energy through your radical chakra, a macros (anorexia) occurs (sometimes in combination with the sacral chakra and solar plexus chakra blockages) in some cases—an escape reaction. However, you will continue to face the problems of "earthly life" until you have learned to accept them as milestones of a comprehensive evolution.

Possibilities of purification and activation of the first chakra

Natural experience

The contemplation of a rising blood-red sun and shimmering dawn or twilight acidifies and harmonizes the radical chakra and unleashes constrained structures that fall within its field of action.

To communicate with the reassuring, stabilizing and uplifting energy of our planet through the first chakra, sit in the position of the loto, or the tailor; on the bare earth and consciously breathe in its smell.

If you can combine both nature experiences with each other, there will be an optimal integral effect on the radical chakra.

Sound therapy

Musical form: Music with monotonous and strongly accented rhythms is ideal for activating the radical chakra. The archaic music of many primitive people best expresses this form of music. Likewise, their dances also aspire to establish the union with nature, its forces and its creatures.

To harmonize the radical chakra, you can use the sounds of nature. In case you don't have the "original sound" at your disposal, these sounds are currently recorded on a multitude of magnetospheric tapes and discs.

Vocal: The radical chakra is assigned the vowel "u." It is sung with the deep C tone of the musical scale. The "u" sound triggers a downward-facing movement in the direction of your roots. It leads you to the depths of the subconscious and activates the original earth energies of the first chakra.

Chromotherapy

The first chakra is activated by a clear and bright red. The red color warms, enlivens, and provides vitality, dynamism and value. When red is mixed with a little blue, it helps you penetrate vital instincts with intellectual strength.

Gemmotherapy

Agate: The agate provides seriousness, endurance and balance. It helps to dissolve negative emotions and protects the inner being. It awakens the evaluation of the body itself and acts constructively on the organs of reproduction. Agate discs with crystalline inclusion introduce a growing life (whether a physical or spiritual child), as well as safety and protection. They provide confidence and facilitate deliveries.

Hematites: Hematites give strength, have an uplifting effect on the body, and mobilize hidden forces. Therefore, they help in states of weakness and provide support for healing after an illness. In addition, they promote a healthy formation of blood and cells.

Blood Jasper: The blood jasper, green and red, binds you with the elemental strength and patient love of the "Mother Earth." It teaches you non-utilitarian character and modesty, strengthens the blood, brings vitality, stability, endurance and patience. It purifies and transforms the physical body, and conveys the feeling of security in the natural cycle of life, from which energy and rest can be created.

Granite: The granite brings active energy, will intensity, self-confidence and success. It opens the view for the occult until you reach clairvoyance. It stimulates sexuality and contributes to modify it in a transformative and constructive force. At the body level, it contributes to diseases of the sex organs and stimulates blood circulation.

Red Coral: Red coral provides fluid vital energy and strength. It has a stimulating and life-giving effect and promotes hematopoiesis. It gives stability, and at the same time favors flexibility, so that you can have self-security while simultaneously following the course of life.

Ruby: Ruby transmits a life-giving, warm and creative energy that leads to clarification and transformation. It establishes a harmonious link between bodily and spiritual love, between sexuality and spirituality, through which new experiential forms are opened.

Aromatherapy

Cedar: The rough aroma of cedar oil unites you with the earthly forces and essences of nature. It helps to collect energy, transmits tranquility and the feeling of security within "Mother Earth."

Spice nail: The smell of spice cloves helps dissolve the stagnant energies in the radical chakra. It favors the willingness to release structures that constrain, arising from the need for delimitation and security, and to be open for new and fresh energies. In this way, it brings transformation and renewal if you let the message of its vibrations enter you.

Forms of yoga that act primarily on the first chakra

Hatha Yoga: Development of consciousness through the purification and stimulation of the body base through certain exercises and physical postures linked to breathing exercises.

Kundalini Yoga: Awakening of the so-called energy of the snake, which runs from the coxal bone parallel to the spine and which, in its ascent, activates and vivifies all other chakras. For this there are different physical and spiritual exercises.

The second chakra and its correspondences

Keywords: Emotions. The change and how I adapt to it. The movement. Pleasure. The desire. Sexuality, orgasm. The protection. Empathy and sociability. Creativity. This place of the body needs to feel acceptance and love for itself that allows it to be its refuge affectionately and positively.

- Location: Below the navel.
- Sanskrit name: Swadhisthana.
- Sound: Vam.
- Phoneme: U
- Verb: Sorry.

- Colors: Orange if you are looking to activate it, blue if you want to calm it down.
- Foods: Liquids.
- Essential oils: Ylang-ylang, sandalwood.
- Gems: All orange, coral, carnelian, opal.
- Corresponding element: Water
- Sensory function: Taste
- Symbol: Six-petal loto
- Basic principle: Creative propagation of being
- Body maps: Pelvic cavity, reproductive organs, kidneys, bladder; all moods;
  such as: blood, lymph, digestive juices, sperm
- Corresponding glands: Sexual organs: ovaries, prostate, testicles. The role of sexual organs is the formation of male and female sexual characteristics and the regulation of the female cycle.

Astrological correspondences:

- Cancer/Moon: Wealth of feelings, sensitivity, fertility
- Pound/Venus: Dedication to you, relationships, sensory, artistic sensitivity.

- Scorpio/Pluto: Sensory ambition, the transformation of personality by overcoming the self in sexual union.

Note: Some writings indicate the spleen chakra as the second chakra. However, such a chakra is an important secondary center that matches its operation with the third chakra. This deviation from the original system has its beginning in the denial of sexuality in some esoteric schools. Subsequently there was sometimes a mixture of the systems, so that today the realm of sexuality is often assigned to the spleen chakra and sometimes to the radical center.

Mission and operation of the second chakra

The second chakra is the center of original unfiltered emotions, sexual energies and creative forces. It is assigned to the water element, from which all biological life has arisen and which in astrology corresponds to the scope of feelings.

Water fertilizes and continually brings about new life in creation. Through the Sacro chakra, we participate in the fertilizing and computing energies that go through all nature. We experience ourselves as part of a perennial creative process that manifests itself in us and, through us, in the form of creative feelings and actions.

The sacred chakra is often regarded as the authentic sensing position of Shakti, the "feminine" aspect of God in the form of creative force. Its field of action includes in the male the organs of procreation, which carry within themselves the impulse for the creation of new life. In women we find here those areas where she receives the creative impulse and brings forth new life, and the place where the new incipient being is protected, fed, and where everything the child needs to prosper is provided.

But the water element also purifies, dissolves and drags how much it is gripped and opposes its flow alive. This is manifested, within the body scope, by the detoxifying and excretory activity of the kidneys and bladder. On an animian plane we live it through liberation and letting feelings flow, so we are willing to experience life always in an original and new way.

Our interpersonal relationships, in particular, those relating to the opposite sex, are decisively marked by the functioning of the second chakra. The multiple varieties of erotic play also belong to their field of action as well as the abandonment of the limited ego and the experience of greater unity through sexual union.

Harmonic operation

Flowing naturally with life and feelings shows the harmonic functioning of an open sacral chakra. You will be open and natural to others, and especially for the opposite sex. The sexual union with a loved one is for you a possibility to enter with your vibrations in the dance of the male and female energies of creation, in order to experience a superior unity with all nature and grow towards an inner integration.

You feel that the flow of life also flows into creation through your body, your soul, and your spirit. Thus, you participate in the deep joy of creation, and life always fills you with wonder and enthusiasm. Your feelings are original—your creative actions. Both bear fruit in your own life, as well as the lives of others.

Harmonic operation

A sacral chakra dysfunction often originates from puberty. Growing sexual forces cause insecurity, as parents and educators are rarely able to provide proper management of these energies. Often, in the earliest childhood, they have also lacked delicacy and body closeness. This can now lead to a denial and rejection of sexuality, so uninhibited expression loses its creative potential and energies manifest inappropriately. This often occurs in the form of sexual fantasies or repressed institute, which make their way in from time to time. Another possible impact is that you use sexuality as a drug. Your creative potential will not be detected here either, and it will deviate. In both cases there are tensions and insecurity against the other sex. Your sensory perception is relatively rude and you have a tendency to put the satisfaction of your sexual needs first.

Perhaps you simply live in a continuous longing for a fulfilling sexual relationship, without realizing that the cause of this desire not being realized lies in yourself.

With the loss of naivety and innocence in dealing with sexual energies, you also lose the candor to express or manifest these energies in creation, for the play of yin and yang forces and, therefore, for childish wonder for the miracle of life.

Hypofunction

The function of the sacral chakra arises in most cases from childhood itself. Your parents probably already suppressed their own sensuality and sexuality, and you lacked sensory stimulation, contacts, caresses and tenderness. The consequence was that you completely retracted your antennas in this area.

Then, in puberty, you completely blocked the sexual energies that struggled to get out. Through your repression "crowned by success" you come to a lack of self-esteem, numbness of emotions and the coldness of sexual feelings. Life seems sad and unworthy of being lived.

Possibilities of purification and activation of the second chakra

Natural experience

Moonlight and contemplation or contact with transparent water in nature activate the second chakra.

The Moon, in particular, the full moon, stimulates your feelings and makes you receptive to the messages of your soul, which want to be transmitted to you in images of fantasy and dreams.

Calm contemplation of a natural and transparent watercourse, a bath in those waters or small sips of a freshwater fountain help you purify the soul, lighten it and free it from emotional blockages and stagnation, so that life can flow in you more freely.

If you can join the contemplation of the moon and contact with the water together, you will have an optimal effect on the second chakra.

Sound therapy

Musical form: Any type of appropriate music is suitable to activate the second chakra, which awakens the carefree joy of living. Also, fluid rhythms and popular and coupled dances enter this therapy. On the other hand, any music that brings out your emotions suffices.

To calm and harmonize the sacral chakra, you can listen to the song of the birds, the murmur of the water flowing in nature, or the singing sound of a small indoor fountain.

Vocal: The radical chakra is activated by a closed "o," just like the first "o" of the word "sofort." It is sung in the rekeying of the scale. The vowel "o" triggers a circular motion. In its closed form, which approaches the "u" sound, it awakens the depth of feelings and leads you to the circular whole, in which yin and yang, the female and male energy, reach unity by the fluid harmony of forces.

In our language, the exclamation "Oh!" expresses an admiration laden with feeling. Similarly, the ability to surprise us by the miracles of creation is enlivened by the sound "o."

Chromotherapy

A light orange color activates the second chakra. Orange conveys a life-giving and renewing energy and releases numb emotional patterns. It promotes a sense of self-esteem and awakens the joy of sensory pleasure. In Ayurveda it is said that orange is the interior color of the water.

Gemmotherapy

Coralline: The coralline unites you with the beauty and creative force of this earth. It helps you live and promotes concentration. It brings back amazement at the miracles of creation, causes life to flow again, and activates the capacity for creative expression.

Moonstone: The moonstone opens you up for your richness of inner feelings. It unites you with your sensitive, receptive and dreamy essential side, and helps you accept and integrate it into your personality. It absorbs the fear of feelings and has a harmonizing effect on emotional balance.

On the body plane, it supports the purification of blocked lymphatic pathways, and in women it is responsible for maintaining an adequate hormonal balance.

Aromatherapy

Ylang-ylang: This refined oil extracted from the flowers of the ylang-ylang tree is one of the best-known aphrodisiacs. It has a relaxing effect and at the same time opens you up to more subtle sensory sensations. Its sweet aroma conveys a sense of security, from which you will re-trust the flow of your feelings. Stagnant or excited emotions are dragged and dissolved.

Sandalwood oil has often been used in the East to increase sexual energies and elevate the union with a loving couple to the plane of a spiritual experience. In addition, it stimulates fantasy and awakens joy for creative action. The vibrations of sandalwood produce the integration of spiritual energies into all planes of our thinking, feeling and acting.

Form of yoga that acts primarily on the second chakra

Tantric Yoga: In tantra all nature is considered as a game of the female and male forces, shakti and Shiva, who in a perpetual creative dance, generate the world of appearances or phenomena.

115

By opening all the senses, by means of complete "yes" to life, and by the use and elevation of sexual experience, tantra aspires to a union with this "cosmic sexuality."

The third chakra and its correspondences

Keywords: The ego. I am. The own territory. Power and will. Energy. The transformation. The personal mind. This place needs to understand the situations that it lives in a clear, direct way and with a certain rational lucidity that flows in harmony with the intuitive mind.

- Location: In the pit of the stomach.
- Sanskrit name: Manipura.
- Sound: Ram.
- Phoneme: A
- Verb: I can.
- Colors: Yellow to activate it and purple to calm it.
- Foods: Cereals.
- Magic with candles: Between the "three wishes" in front of the birthday cake and conscious meditation.

- Essential oils: Lavender, rosemary, bergamot, sage, carnation, cinnamon, daisy, sunflower.
- Gems: All yellow, topaz, citrine, amber.
- Corresponding element: Fire.
- Sensory function: View.
- Symbol: Ten-petty loto.
- Basic principle: Configuration of the being.
- Body correspondences: Lower back, abdominal cavity, digestive system, stomach, liver, spleen, gallbladder; vegetative nervous system.
- Corresponding gland: Pancreas (liver).

The pancreas plays a decisive role in the processing and digestion of food. It produces the hormone insulin, which is important for the balance of blood sugar and for the metabolism of carbohydrates. Enzymes secreted by the pancreas are important for the metabolism of fats and proteins.

Astrological correspondences:

- Leo/Sun: Heat, strength, fullness, aspiration for recognition, power and social position.
- Sagittarius/Jupiter: Affirming vital experiences, growth and enlargement, synthesis, wisdom, integration.

- Virgo/Mercury: Subdivision, analysis, adaptation, selfless or altruistic service.
- Mars: Energy, activity, disposition for action, the imposition of one's personality.

Mission and operation of the third chakra

The third chakra finds different denominations. There are also different indications of where it sits. It is the main chakra and several secondary chakras that, however, intertwine so closely in their functioning that all of them can be considered together as a main chakra.

Thus, the third chakra has a complex scope of functions. It is assigned to the fire element; fire means light, heat, energy and activity; and on the spiritual plane, also purification.

The solar plexus chakra represents our Sun, our energy center. Here we absorb the energy of the Sun, which among other functions has to feed our etheric body, also nourishing the physical body with vitality and sustaining it. In the third chakra we enter into an active relationship with the things of the world and with other people. It's the area from which our emotional energy flows out. Our interpersonal relationships, sympathies and antipathies, and the ability to establish lasting emotional bonds are broadly governed from this center.

For the ordinary man, the third chakra is the personality seat. It is the place where he finds his social identification and tries to confirm himself by personal strength, the will for performance and the aspiration of power, or by adapting to social norms.

An important function of the third chakra is to purify the instincts and desires of the lower chakras, to consciously direct and use their creative energy, as well as to manifest in the material world the spiritual fullness of the upper chakras, and achieve a degree of maximum consummation in life at all levels.

It is found in direct union with the astral body, also called the body of desire or ambition, and which is the bearer of our emotions. The vital impulses, desires and feelings of the lower chakras are deciphered here, "digested," transforming into higher energy before being used in conjunction with the energies of the higher chakras for the conscious configuration of our lives.

We can find a corresponding principle in the physical plane in the liver area. In conjunction with the digestive system, the liver has the function of analyzing the food ingested, separating the useless from the profitable, and transforming the user into usable substances, transporting them to the right places in the body.

The conscious affirmation and integration of feelings and desires and our life experiences lead to the détente and openness of the third chakra, with which light continually grows in us and our life, and our world become increasingly enlightened.

Our general mood depends very intensely on how much light we let into us. We feel enlightened, cheerful and satisfied inside when the third chakra is open; on the contrary, our mood is unbalanced and bleak when blocked or deranged. This feeling is continually projected into the outside world, so that all life can seem enlightened or dark. The amount of light within us determines the clarity of our vision and the quality of what we contemplate.

The increasing integration and inner totality cause the yellow light of intellectual understanding to gradually transform into the third chakra into the golden light of wisdom and fullness.

With the solar plexus chakra, we also perceive the vibrations of other people directly, and then we react accordingly to the quality of such vibrations. When faced with negative vibrations, here we often experience imminent danger. We recognize this because the third chakra is contracted unintentionally, as a temporary protection mechanism. However, it becomes superfluous when the light within us is so large that it radiates intensely outward and surrounds our body as with a protective envelope.

Harmonic operation

When the third chakra is open and works harmoniously, a feeling of peace, inner harmony with yourself, with life and your position before it, is transmitted. You can accept yourself with all your being and you are able to respect the feelings and peculiarities of other people.

You have the natural ability to accept feelings, desires and vital experiences, to recognize their function for your evolution, to see them "in the right light" and to integrate them into your personality in a way that leads you to totality.

Your action spontaneously comes into line with natural laws that are effective throughout the universe and in man's own. As it encourages evolution, it helps to open wealth and fullness for you and your fellow people, both indoors and outdoors. You're full of light and strength. The clarity in you also surrounds your body: this protects you from negative vibrations and radiates throughout your environment.

In combination with an open front and coronal chakra, you detect that everything visible is composed of different vibrations of light. Your desires are fulfilled spontaneously, since you are so closely bound with the luminous force of all things you attract like a magnet as desired.

Thus you realize in your life the knowledge that fulness is your right acquired at birth and your divine inheritance.

When the third chakra has a strong one-sided accent and dysfunction, you would like to influence everything according to your sense, control both your inner world and your outside world, as well as exercise power and conquer. But you find yourself driven by inner uneasiness and dissatisfaction. You've probably experienced little recognition in your childhood and youth. You have not possessed any true sense of self-esteem, and now you seek in the outer life that confirmation and satisfaction that have always been lacking inwardly. To do this, you develop a huge impulse of activity, with which you try to cover the corrosive feeling of insufficiency. You lack inner serenity, and you find it hard to free yourself and unwind.

Since you believe you are predominantly destined to gain recognition and external wealth, you will probably succeed.

The position that everything is feasible leads to the control and repression of "vicious" and unwanted feelings. Consequently, your emotions will stagnate. However, from time to time they will break that wall moved by rejection and control and will flood you without you being able to steer them properly. In addition, you exasperate easily, and in your excitability there is a lot of that anger that you have swallowed over time without processing it.

Finally, you must note that the mere aspiration for external wealth and recognition cannot give you any lasting satisfaction.

Hypofunction

When there is poor functioning of the third chakra you often feel defeated and unencouraged.

You see obstacles everywhere that oppose the fulfillment of your wishes.

The free development of your personality was probably strongly hampered as a child. For fear of losing recognition from your parents or educators, you have almost completely retracted the manifestation of your feelings and swallowed many things you weren't able to digest. Thus, "emotional slags" have been formed that mitigate the fiery energy of the solar plexus chakra and take away the force and spontaneity of your desires and actions.

Even today you try to gain recognition through adaptation, which leads to rejection and poor integration of vital desires and emotions. In difficult situations, you're invaded by a languid sensation in your stomach or you get so nervous that your actions are fickle and uncoordinated.

What you'd like most is to shut yourself down to new challenges. The unused experiences cause you distress, and you don't really believe in what's meant by a life struggle.

Possibilities of purification and activation of the third chakra

Natural experience

The golden light of the sun corresponds to the light, heat and force of the solar plexus chakra. If you consciously open yourself up to their influence, these qualities will be activated in you.

The observation of a field of rapeseed or cereal ripe and resplendent by the sun also transmits to you the experience of the fullness manifested as resonance, caused by the heat and the luminous force of the sun.

In the center of the sunflower, in the unit of the moving circle, you find the moving spiral pattern, and on the petals, the golden light radiating outward. By imbuing yourself in it, the pattern of this natural mandala you experience in the inner experience of unity, there is a movement and activity full of meaning, orderly and at the same time dancers, who radiate outward with energy, joy, softness and absolute beauty.

Sound therapy

Musical form: The third chakra is activated by fiery rhythms. Orchestral music, with its harmonic conjunction of a lot of sounds, can be used to harmonize the solar plexus chakra. In the case of hyperactivity, any relaxing music that leads you to your center is suitable to reassure you.

Vocal: The solar plexus chakra is assigned an open "o," as the second "o" of the word "sofort". Here too, the "o" causes a circular motion that is directed outward through the "o" opening. It favors the exterior configuration of the being from an interior whole. The open "o" approaches the "a" of the heart chakra. It provides breadth, fullness and joy in manifestation.

Chromotherapy

A light and sunny yellow activates and intensifies the functioning of the third chakra. Yellow accelerates nerve activity and thinking, and encourages contact and exchange with others. It counteracts a feeling of inner fatigue, joviality and serene ease. When you're in a passive or dreamy state, a light yellow will help you get actively into life. In addition, it promotes physical digestion and 'psychic digestion.'

The chromatic hue of golden yellow has a clarifying and sedative effect on psychic problems and diseases. It enhances intellectual activities and promotes that form of wisdom that is born only of experience.

Gemmotherapy

Tiger's Eye: The tiger's eye favors both exterior and inner visual ability. It sharpens understanding and helps you recognize your mistakes and act accordingly.

Amber: Amber provides warmth and confidence. Its solar strength leads you on your way to greater joy and clearer light. It conveys intuition to you and tells you how you can perform in life. In this way, amber gives you a lucky hand in the various companies you undertake.

On the body plane, it purifies the body, has a balancing effect on the digestive and hormonal system and purifies and enhances the liver.

Topaz: Golden yellow topaz fills you with flowing energy and warm sunlight. It brings greater awareness, wakefulness, clarity, joy and vivacity. It also eliminates the feelings of ballast and murky thoughts: an aid to anxieties and depression.

It strengthens and stimulates the whole body and promotes spiritual and body digestion.

Citrine: Citrine transmits well-being, warmth, vivacity, safety and confidence. It helps you process life experiences and integrates them into your personality, as well as apply intuitive perceptions in everyday life. It provides fullness, both indoors and outdoors, and supports you in the realization of your goals.

In the physical field, it favors the excretion or elimination of toxins and helps in digestive disorders and diabetes. It also activates blood and boosts nerve activity.

Aromatherapy

Lavender: The essence of lavender has a sedative and relaxing effect on a third hyperactive chakra. Its soft and warm vibrations help in the dissolution and processing of stagnant emotions.

Romero: The essence of rosemary, aromatic and rough, is particularly suitable in case of hypofunction of the solar plexus chakra. It has a life-giving and stimulating effect, helps overcome laziness and encourages the willingness to do so.

Bergamot: The vibrations of the oil that is extracted from the fruits of the bergamot tree contain a lot of light. Its fresh and lemony aroma enhances our vital energies. It gives us self-confidence.

A form of yoga that acts primarily on the third chakra.

Karmic yoga: In karmic yoga we aspire to altruism in action, without thinking about the fruits and personal results of actions. In this way the karmic yogi opens himself to the divine will and concordats his actions with the natural forces of evolution, which reflect God's will for creation.

The fourth chakra and its correspondences

Keywords: Unconditional love, compassion, affinity, relationships, healing, breathing, devotion, the bridge. It is the center of love where we interact affectively with partners, children, family, colleagues, or friends. You need to give and receive love in all types of relationships where love is possible.

- Location: Heart.
- Sanskrit name: Anahata.
- Sound: Lam.
- Phoneme: E
- Verb: I love it.
- Colors: Green and pink to activate it, intense green to calm it.
- Foods: Vegetables.
- Essential oils: Roses, jasmine, marjoram.
- Gems: All green or pink, green quartz, rose, rhodochrosite, moonstone.
- Corresponding element: Air.
- Sensory function: Touch.

- Symbol: 12-petal loto. (a)
- Basic principle: Delivery of being.
- Body correspondences: Heart, upper back with the rib cage and chest cavity, the lower area of the lungs, blood and circulatory system, skin.
- Corresponding gland: Timo. The thymus regulates growth and controls the lymphatic system. In addition, it has the mission of stimulating and strengthening the immune system.

Astrological correspondences:

- Leo/Sun: Sentimental warmth, cordiality, generosity.
- Pound/Venus: Contact, love, aspiration to harmony, complementation in the "you."
- Saturn: Overcoming the individual ego, essential for selfless love.

CHAPTER 9

MISSION AND OPERATION OF THE FOURTH CHAKRA

The fourth chakra forms the central point of the chakra system. It links the three physical-emotional lower centers with the three psychic-spiritual upper centers. Its symbol is the hexagon, which represents very intuitively how the energies of the three upper and three lower chakras penetrate each other. The fourth chakra is assigned the element air and sense of touch. This signals the mobility of the heart, the movement towards something, the contact, the letting go, the being in contact with things. We find here the ability to emphasize and "feel with," to balance moods and to go into resonance with vibrations. Through this center, we also perceive the beauty of nature and the harmony of music, graphic art and poetry. Here, images, words and sounds are transformed into feelings.

The mission of the cordial chakra is the union for love. Every cripple of intimate contact, uniqueness, harmony and love is manifested through the cordial chakra, even when we come out in its form of sadness, pain, or anguish at the separation or loss of love.

In its purified and completely open form, the cordial chakra is the center of true and unconditional love, a love that only exists on its own, that cannot be had or lost. In combination with the higher chakras, this love becomes Bhakti, in divine love, and leads to knowledge of divine presence throughout creation, to uniqueness with the most intimate nucleus, with the heart of all things of the universe. The path of the heart towards this goal passes through "yes," full of love and understanding, towards ourselves as a premise for the "yes" to others and to life.

If through the third chakra and knowledge we have accepted that all life experiences, desires and emotions have a deeper meaning, and through it and the associated learning mission, we want to return to a broader order, we will find in the room chakra a loving acceptance emanating from the knowledge of the heart that all feelings and all manifestations of life have originally arisen from the longing of love, of union with life and, therefore, are ultimately a manifestation of love.

With every union, we generate separation and negativity. The positive and loving "yes" generates, on the other hand, a vibration in which negative forms and feelings, which dissolve, cannot be maintained and manifest. You may have already experienced the fact that an intense feeling of sadness, anger, or despair has been neutralized when you have dedicated your loving attention, without prejudice and integrity to that feeling. Try it some time.

When we suffer from difficulties or illness, we can see that, through loving dedication to the diseased organ or the part of the sick body, we can greatly accelerate healing.

In this way, through the cordial chakra, we have a great potential for transformation and healing: both for ourselves and for others. Love for ourselves, the acceptance of our whole essence from the depths of our hearts, can transform and heal us fundamentally. And it is a premise for a satisfying love for others, for "feeling with," for understanding and the deep joy of living.

The cordial chakra is a center whose force radiates with a particular intensity to the outside. An open, cordial chakra will have a spontaneous healing and transformative effect on other people (on the other hand, in a consciously applied healing activity the frontal chakra is also involved).

The cordial chakra radiates in the colors green and pink, and sometimes also in gold. Green is the color of healing, as well as harmony and sympathy. When an aura seer perceives, in a person's cordial chakra, a light and luminous green, it is for him an indication of a very marked healing ability. A golden aura, or with pink iridescent, indicates a person who lives in pure love and fully devoted to the divine.

Often, the chakra of the heart is called the door to the soul, since not only do our deepest and most vivid feelings of love settle in it, but through this energy center, we can also come into contact with the universal part of our soul, with the divine sparks in us. It also plays a decisive role in the refinement of perception, which is paired with the opening of the front chakra, the so-called third eye, since it is the delivery that makes us sensitive to the subtler realms of creation. This means that, in parallel with the development of the cordial chakra, the higher faculties of the frontal chakra are developed.

For this reason, many spiritual disciplines, both East and West, have specifically focused on the opening of the cordial chakra.

Harmonic operation

When your cordial chakra is completely open and interacts harmoniously with the plus chakras, you become a channel of divine love. The energies of your heart can transform your world and unite the people around you, reconcile them and heal them. You radiate a natural warmth, cordiality and joviality that opens the hearts of your fellow citizens, awakens confidence and gives joy. Sharing feelings and a willingness to help are not over-the-top for you.

Your feelings are free from internal turmoil and conflict, doubts and uncertainties. You love for love itself from the joy of giving, without expecting anything in return. And you feel safe and at home in all creation. All in all, in what you do, "you put your whole heart."

The love of your heart also purifies your perception, so that you also perceive the cosmic play of separation and the new union in all manifestations of any plane of creation, a cosmic game that is ported and penetrated by divine love and harmony. You yourself have experienced that from the separation of the universal and divine aspect of life, and the suffering resulting from it is the longing for reunification with the divine. And that only through this prior separation can the conscious and complete experience of the love of God and the infinite joy in him come about.

You observe the events of the world from this wisdom of the heart, and you observe your life in a new light.

The love of your heart spontaneously supports all the aspirations that make love for God and his creation grow. You know that the whole life of creation lives in your heart. You no longer contemplate life from the outside as something separate from you, but as if it were a part of your own life.

The feeling of vivacity in you is so great that only now do you really know what "life" means in its original form: a permanent expression of divine love and glory.

Dysfunction of the heart chakra can be expressed in several ways: for example, you would like to give, always be there for others without having to be at the source of love. In secret (perhaps without being aware of it or without confessing to yourself) you still expect to receive recognition and confirmation in exchange for all your "love," and you are disappointed when your efforts are not sufficiently rewarded.

Either you feel powerful and strong and give others your strength, or you are not able to accept love yourself, to open yourself to receive. The tender and gentle will bewilder you. Maybe you'll tell yourself you don't need the love of others. This posture is often paired with a "ufano" chest, an indication of the internal armor and rejection of pain and attacks.

Hypofunction

The poor functioning of the cordial chakra makes you easily vulnerable and dependent on the love and sympathy of others. When you are rejected, you feel deeply affected; just when, for once, you had the courage to open up? Then you retract back into your shell, you're sad and depressed. It is true that you would want to give love, but for fear of a new rejection, you do not find the right way to do it, which affirms you again and again of your incapacity.

Possibly, you also try to compensate for your lack of love in a particular friendship, bringing you joy in a rather impersonal way to everyone alike, without letting yourself, however, introduce yourself deeper into people. But as soon as it really appeals to your heart, you react evasively for fear of a possible wound.

When your cordial chakra is completely closed, it manifests itself in dryness and disinterest, which can reach the "coldness of heart." In order to even feel something, you need a strong external stimulation. You're decompensated and suffering from depression.

Possibilities of purification and activation of the fourth chakra

Natural experience

Any silent walk through the green and untouched nature harmonizes our whole being through the cordial chakra. Any flower conveys to us the message of love and innocent joy and lets the same qualities flourish in our hearts. The red flowers are particularly suitable for gently activating and healing the energies of the cordial chakra.

A pink-tinged sky with delicate cloud formations lifts and widens the heart. Let yourself be wrapped and carried by the beauty and softness of colors and shapes of this image of the sky.

Sound therapy

Musical form: Any classical music, "New Age" music or sacred music, both eastern and western tradition, which makes your heart dance along with life and creation, and awakens the heart force of love in your chakra, has a life-giving and harmonizing effect on it. Also, sacred or meditative dances, in their movements, manifest the harmony and joy of creation.

Vocal: The cordial chakra is assigned the vowel "a." Used in the scale f key. The "a" symbolizes the sudden discovery of the heart, as manifested in our exclamation "ah!" It is the most open sound of all, representing the greatest possible fullness in the manifestation of the human voice. In the "a" lies the unprejudiced acceptance of all events, acceptance from which love is born. It is also the most frequent vowel of babies, who's intellect cannot distinguish between "good" and "evil," when they "comment" on their experiences.

Chromotherapy

Green: The color of the meadows and forests of our planet provides harmony and empathy, gives us a conciliatory spirit, makes us feel sympathy and transmits to us a feeling of peace. It also has a regenerative effect on the body, spirit and soul, and brings new energies.

Pink: The soft, delicate vibrations of pink dissolve heart spasms. They arouse feelings of love and tenderness and provide a childish feeling of happiness. In addition, they stimulate creative activity.

Gemmotherapy

Pink quartz: The delicate and pinkish light of pink quartz favors softness, tenderness and love. It envelops your soul in a loving vibration in which they can heal the wounds of the heart caused by hardness, brutality or inattention, and can open your soul more and more to love and give it more love.

Pink quartz teaches you to love and accept yourself, open your heart to the manifestation of love and sweetness that is in you, in other people and in creation. It also makes you sensitive to the beauty of music, poetry, painting and other arts, and stimulates your fantasy and your ability to express creative expression.

Tourmaline: Pink-red tourmaline takes you out of indolent sentimental structures; opens and widens your heart. It also opens your conscience to the joyful and jovial aspect of love. It joins you with the feminine manifestation of divine love, which is expressed in the beauty of creation, in carefree joviality, in spiritual dance and in the game. In this way it integrates the different manifestations of worldly and divine love.

Pink tourmaline with a green flange is also particularly suitable for the cordial chakra, which is often cut into discs (watermelon tourmaline). Here, the qualities of pink-red tourmaline are embedded in the healing and harmonizing vibration of green.

Kunzite: In the kunzite are joined the delicate rose of superior love and the violet of the coronal chakra, which supports unification with the divine.

The kunzite opens your cordial chakra to divine love. It helps you grow your heart's love for altruism and perception. To do this, it provides guidance and always takes you back this way.

Emerald: Emerald is the love of the universe, since it intensifies and deepens love in all planes. It gives peace and harmony and puts you in harmony with the forces of nature. It also challenges you to make yourself equal to its radiant light and shows you the areas where it doesn't happen yet.

The emerald attracts healing energies from the cosmos in the direction of Earth. Regenerate, rejuvenate, refresh and reassure.

Jade: The soft green light of jade provides peace, harmony, the wisdom of heart, justice and modesty. The jade relaxes and calms the heart, makes you discover and live the beauty of everything created, thus fostering your esteem and love for creation. The jade helps in the face of restlessness and bewilderment, and encourages the reconciliation of peaceful sleep and pleasant dreams.

Aromatherapy

Rose Essence: There is no other aroma that has such a strong harmonizing effect above all our being as the precious essence of roses. Its delicate and loving vibrations mitigate and heal the wounds of our hearts. They awaken perception by the manifestation of love, beauty and harmony throughout creation. They reinstitute in the heart a deep joy and willingness for dedication. The essence of roses also causes stimulation and refinement of sensory joys, at the same time promoting their transformation for supra-personal love.

Form of yoga that acts primarily on the fourth chakra

Yoga Bhakti: Bhakti yoga is the way that leads to the love of God and gives it to the individual for fulfillment in God. The bhakta deepens and intensifies his feelings and turns him to God. Everything he means, he sees it in all things and rises in love for Him.

The fifth chakra and its correspondences

Keywords: Sound, communication, creativity, creation, symbol ideas, telepathy, the media.

Harmonize with the divine will within, commit to telling the truth. You need to express your truth.

- Location: Throat.
- Sanskrit name: Vishudha.
- Sound: Ham.
- Phoneme: i
- Verb: I speak.
- Corresponding element: Ether.
- Sensory function: Ear.
- Symbol: 16-petal loto.
- Basic principle: Resonance with being.
- Body maps: Neck area, cervical area, chin area, ears, speech apparatus (voice), respiratory ducts, bronchi, the upper area of the lungs, esophagus, arms.
- Colors: Sky blue and turquoise to activate it, fuchsia to calm it.
- Gems: Turquoise, Aquamarine, Celestine, Blue Lace Agate.
- Foods: fresh and dried fruits.
- Essential oils: Sage, eucalyptus, frankincense, benzoin.

Corresponding gland: Thyroid.

The thyroid plays an important role in the growth of the skeleton and internal organs. It is responsible for the balance between physical and psychic growth and regulates metabolism, that is, the way and speed in which we transform our food into energy and in which we consume such energy. It also regulates iodine metabolism and calcium balance in the blood and tissues.

Astrological correspondences:

- **Gemini/Mercury:** Communication, exchange of knowledge and experiences.
- **Mars:** Active self-manifestation.
- **Taurus/Venus:** Sense of space and form.
- **Aquarius/Uranus:** Divine inspiration, the transmission of wisdom and superior knowledge, independence.

Mission and operation of the fifth chakra

In the neck chakra, we find the center of human expression capacity, communication and inspiration. It is attached to a smaller secondary chakra, which is seated at the back of the neck and opens backward. Also these two energy centers are often considered as a single chakra. In its functioning, however, the cervical chakra is so closely linked with the neck chakra that we have integrated it into the interpretation of the latter.

The fifth chakra also forms an important union of the lower chakras with the centers of the head. It serves as a bridge between our thinking and our feeling, between our impulses and the reactions we have to them, and simultaneously transmits the contents of all chakras to the outside world. Through the neck chakra we manifest all that lives in us, our laughter and our weeping, our feelings of love and joy or anguish and anger, our intentions and desires, and also our ideas, intuitions and perception of the inner worlds.

The element that is assigned to the neck chakra is the ether. In the doctrine of yoga, it is considered the fundamental element from which the elements of the lower chakras are formed by compaction: earth, water, fire, air. But the ether is also the bearer of the sound, of the spoken word, and of the word of the creator; it is, in short, the transmitter of information on all planes.

Thus, the communication of our inner life to the outside is predominantly through spoken word, but also through our mimicry, and through other creative manifestations, such as music, graphic art and interpretive dance, etc. The creativity we found in the sacral chakra is joined in the neck chakra with the energies of the remaining chakras, and the forming power of the ether gives it a certain figure that we relay to the outside world.

However, we can only express what we find in ourselves. Thus, through the fifth chakra, we first receive the faculty of self-reflection. The premise necessary to be able to reflect is a certain inner distance. As we develop the neck chakra, we are more and more aware of our mental body, and we can separate its functioning from the functioning of the emotional body, the etheric body and the physical body. This means that our thoughts are no longer the hostages of our physical feelings and sensations, so objective knowledge is possible.

The ether is also defined as space (Akasha), in which the most compact elements deploy their effectiveness. The deepest knowledge is conferred upon us when we are open and unobstructed as infinite space, as the wide sky (whose light blue color is the color of the neck chakra), when we remain silent and listen attentively to the interior space and outside. The sensory function of the ear is associated with the fifth chakra. Here we open our ears, listen attentively to the hidden or unhidden voices of creation. We also perceive our own inner voice, come into contact with the spirit inherent in us, and receive its inspiration. And we develop unwavering confidence in the superior personal guide. We are also aware of our authentic role in life, of our dharma. We know that our own inner worlds are both the non-material planes of life and the outside world, and we are able to collect and relay information from the non-material areas and the higher dimensions of reality. This divine inspiration becomes a carrier of our self-manifestation.

Thus, in the fifth chakra we find our individual expression of perfection in all planes.

Harmonic operation

With a completely open neck chakra, you express clearly and without fear your inner feelings, thoughts and knowledge. You are also able to reveal your weaknesses and show your strengths. Your inner sincerity in front of yourself and in front of others is also expressed in your sincere attitude.

You have the ability to express yourself in a totally creative way with your whole being. But you can also remain silent when it is the right thing to do, and you have the gift of listening to others with your heart and with inner understanding. Your language is full of fantasy and, at the same time, it is very clear to transmit your intention in the most effective way to provoke a fulfillment of your desires. This voice is full. In the face of difficulties and resistance, you remain true to yourself, and you can also say "no" when you think so. You don't let yourself be convinced or dragged by other people's opinions, and instead you retain your independence, freedom and self-determination. Your absence of prejudice and your inner breadth make you open to the reality of non-material dimensions. From here you receive, through the inner voice, information that leads you on your way through life, and you give yourself full confidence to this guide.

You recognize that all phenomena of creation have their own message. They tell you about their own life, their role in the great cosmic game and their aspiration to totality and light. You can communicate with beings from other existential realms, and the knowledge you receive from it, you sensibly relay to your fellow citizens without fearing their judgment. All the creative means of expression you use have the ability to transmit wisdom and truth.

From your inner independence and the free manifestation of your whole being, deep joy and a feeling of fullness and integrity are born in you.

When the energies of your neck chakra are blocked, the understanding between the "head" and the "body" is altered. This can manifest itself in two ways. Either you find it difficult to reflect on your feelings, and you often express your accumulated emotions through thoughtless actions; or you have encapsulated yourself in your intellectuality or your rationalism, you deny the right to life, and the wisdom of your sentimental world only allows you to pass the filter of your self-judgment to very crowded emotions, not allowing them to crash against the judgments of your fellow men. Unconscious feelings of guilt and anxieties prevent you from seeing yourself and showing yourself as you are and freely expressing your innermost thoughts, feelings, and needs. Instead, you try to disguise them with all sorts of words and gestures, behind which you hide your true self.

Your language is either unprocessed and rude, or even objective and cold. You'll probably stutter too. Your voice is relatively loud, and your words have no greater depth of content.

You don't allow yourself to give a weak appearance, you try to look strong at any price. In this way, you put yourself under pressure with demands imposed by yourself. It can also happen that the functions that life imposes on you at some point are too great a burden on your shoulders. Then, you arm yourself in your "scapular waist": you shrug your neck unconsciously to protect yourself from increased efforts, or arm yourself for a new "attack."

An inharmonic functioning of the fifth chakra is also found in people who abuse their word and their ability to express to manipulate their congeners, or who try through uninterrupted eloquence and loquacity to attract attention to themselves.

In general, people whose energies are stagnant in the neck chakra do not have access to the non-material dimensions of being, since they lack candor, inner amplitude and independence, which are the premises for the perception of these areas.

However, there is also the possibility here that you may have deep inner knowledge, but that, out of fear of the judgment of others or out of anguish at isolation, you do not dare to live and manifest them. Since they struggle to manifest themselves, spontaneous poetry, images or the like can arise from there.

Spiritual energies can also become stuck in the head. So its transforming force hardly finds access to your emotions, and the energies of the lower chakras do not give those of the superiors the necessary strength and stability to impose themselves, to realize in your life the inner spirituality.

Hypofunction

Also, in the case of hypofunction, you will have difficulty showing, manifesting and representing yourself. However, here you retract completely, you are preferably shy, quiet and withdrawn, or you talk only about things that are unimportant in your outside life.

However, when you have to externalize something you think or feel in the most intimate, you are easily tied up in your throat and your voice sounds coerced. More often than not in the case of inharmonic functioning, we find here the symptom of stuttering. You are unsure of other people and you fear the judgment they may make about you. So you're intensely oriented towards their opinions and often don't really know what you want yourself. You have no access to the messages of your mind and no confidence in your intuitive powers.

When in the course of life, the fifth chakra has not developed, a certain rigidity appears. The framework drawn by yourself, within which you pass your existence and in which you express your potential, is very small, because you only consider as reality the outside world.

151

Possibilities of purification and activation of the fifth chakra

Natural experience

The clear blue of a clear sky evokes a resonance in your neck chakra. To fully embrace it in you, it is best that you lie relaxed outdoors and open your inner self to the infinite spaciousness of the celestial vault. You will notice how your spirit opens and becomes transparent and how any narrowness or stiffness in your neck chakra and irradiation scope gradually dissolves. You will be inwardly willing to receive the "heavenly messages."

The reflection of the blue sky in a crystal clear course of water also has the effect of expanding and releasing your feelings. The slight murmur of the waves carries the messages of your emotions and sensations hidden up to your conscious. Let yourself be completely penetrated by the vibrating energy of the sky and water, and spirit and feelings will unite in a complementary force.

Sound therapy

Musical form: Music and singing rich in superior tones, as well as sacred and meditative dances accompanied by singing, will act with a hugely life-giving effect on the neck chakra. To harmonize and relax the fifth chakra, the most effective music is the "New Age" with acoustic effects. It provides release and spaciousness and opens the inner ear.

Vocal: The vowel "e" activates the neck chakra. It sings into the sun key of the scale. If your voice slowly goes from an "a" to an "i," at any given moment the "e" sound will emerge. Just as the neck represents a bonding channel between the head and the rest of the body, the "e" of the neck chakra unites the heart and understanding, "a" and "i," and channels its forces outward. As you sing the "e", you will notice that this sound demands maximum pressure from the voice and strengthens the energy of the ex-pressure in your fifth chakra.

Chromotherapy

A light, transparent blue is assigned to the neck chakra. This color fosters tranquility and spaciousness and opens you up for spiritual inspiration.

Gemmotherapy

Aquamarine: The luminous blue color of aquamarine is like the sea in which a clear sky is reflected. Aquamarine helps the soul become a mirror for the infinite breadth of the spirit. It promotes communication with the innermost self and brings light and transparency to the most hidden Ancones of the soul. Its vibrations bring to the soul purity, freedom and breadth, so that it can be opened to visionary clairvoyance and an intuitive understanding, and also helps to express this knowledge freely and creatively. Under the influence of aquamarine, the soul can become a channel for selfless love and healing force.

Turquoise: Turquoise, the color in which the blue of the sky and the green of the earth come together, combines the high ideals of the spirit with the original strength of our planet. It helps to express intellectual ideas and knowledge and integrate them into life on Earth. In addition, it attracts positive energies and protects the body and soul from negative influences.

Chalcedony: White and blue chalcedony has a positive effect on the thyroid gland. It has a sedative and balancing influence on mood, and reduces irritability and hypersensitivity. Thanks to its sedative influence, it opens access to inner inspiration and promotes self-manifestation through language and writing.

Aromatherapy

Sage: The fresh and rough aroma of sage sends healing vibrations to the "language dwelling area." It dissolves the convulsive contractions of the neck chakra, so that our words are expressed harmoniously and vigorously, and can transmit in the most effective way possible, the intention of our soul.

Eucalyptus: The refreshing aroma of eucalyptus brings transparency and breadth to the scope of the fifth chakra. Its vibrations open us for inner inspiration and give us self-manifestation, originality and creativity.

Form of yoga that acts primarily on the fifth chakra

Mantric Yoga: Mantras are meditative syllables that reflect in their specific form of vibration certain aspects of the divine. In Mantric yoga, mantras are repeated mentally uninterruptedly, recited high or sung. In doing so, the vibration of the mantra gradually transforms the practitioner's thought and feeling and resonates with the cosmic and divine power manifested in the mantra.

One exception is transcendental meditation. In this form of meditation, a technique is taught, with whose help the mantra is experienced in planes of consciousness less and less material and subtle, until the meditator overcomes even the most subtle aspect of the mantra, and transcends and reaches the experience of being Pure. This process is consumed several times during each meditation.

The sixth chakra and its correspondences

Keywords: Sight, intuition, clairvoyance, image, knowing, perceiving, insight, mastering, visualization, time, completing the karmic teaching of this life. Divine love and spiritual ecstasy. You need to live the personal experience of spirituality and unconditional love.

- Location: Slightly above the eyes, in the center of the forehead.
- Sanskrit name: Ajna.
- Sound: Om.
- Phoneme: M or N
- Verb: I see.
- Colors: Ultramarine blue, indigo to activate it, to calm it, pale blue.
- Foods: none.
- Essential oils: Mint, jasmine, mugwort, anise, saffron, lavender.
- Sensory function: All senses, also in the form of extrasensory perception.
- Symbols: 96-petal loto (twice 48 petals).
- Basic principle: Knowledge of being.
- Body correspondences: Face; eyes, ears, nose, sinuses, cerebellum, central nervous system.

- Corresponding gland: Pituitary gland (hypothesis).
- Gems: All blue or violet, lapis lazuli, amethyst, fluorite.

The pituitary gland is also sometimes referred to as the master gland, since, through its internal secretive activity, it controls the functioning of all other glands. Like a conductor, it establishes harmonic conjunction of the remaining glands.

Astrological correspondences:

- Mercury: Intellectual knowledge, rational thinking.
- Sagittarius/Jupiter: Holistic thinking, knowledge of internal relations.
- Aquarius/Uranus: Thought of divine inspiration, superior intuition, sudden knowledge.
- Pisces/Neptune: Ability to imagine, intuition, access (through delivery) to inner truths.

Mission and operation of the sixth chakra

Through the sixth chakra the conscious perception of being is consumed. It sets the superior psychic force, the intellectual capacity for differentiation, the capacity of remembrance and will; and on a physical level is the supreme command center of the central nervous system.

Its true color is light indigo, but yellow and violet nuances can also be detected. These colors indicate their different ways of functioning on different planes of consciousness. Rational or intellectual thinking can bring about yellow radiation here; transparent dark blue points to intuition and comprehensive knowledge processes. Extrasensory perception is shown in a violet hue.

Any realization in our lives presupposes thoughts and ideas that can be fed by unconscious emotional patterns, but also by the knowledge of reality. Through the third eye, we are united with the process of manifestation through force of thought. Everything that manifests itself in creation exists in pure and unmanifested form, similar to how in a latent state seed all the information from which the plant will arise is already contained. Quantum physics calls this area the unified field or the realm of the least excitation of matter.

The process of creation begins when the latent being itself becomes aware of its own existence. Then a first subject-object relationship arises, and with it the first duality. The amorphous being adopted a first manifest vibration pattern.

Based on this photo vibration, new differentiated vibration patterns are continually emerging through further awareness processes.

In us, men, are contained all the planes of creation, from pure being to compact matter, and are represented by the different planes of vibration of the chakras. Thus, the process of manifestation is consummated in us and through us.

Since the third eye serves as a seat for all the processes of awareness, here we obtain the power of manifestation until the materialization and dematerialization of matter. We can create new realities on the psychic plane and dissolve old realities.

However, in general, this process does not occur automatically and without conscious action. Most of the thoughts that determine our lives are controlled by our unreleased emotional patterns, and programmed by both our own and others' judgments and prejudices. In this way, often our spirit is not the one who dominates, but the servant of our thoughts laden with emotions, which can partially dominate us.

But these thoughts are also realized in our lives, for what we perceive and live outside is always and ultimately a manifestation of our subjective reality.

With the development of our consciousness and the growing opening of the third eye we can always consciously direct this process. Our power of imagination then generates the energy to fulfill an idea or a desire. Along with an open cordial chakra, we can now also emit healing energies and perform healings remotely.

At the same time, we receive access to all the planes of creation that lie behind physical reality. The knowledge of them comes to us in the form of intuition, through clairvoyant vision or through auditory or tactile clairvoyance. What we may have previously blundered vaguely now becomes a clear perception.

Harmonic operation

In our time there are very few people whose third eye is completely open, since their development always has a development of advanced consciousness. But here the phenomenon that the sixth chakra works harmoniously even if it is not fully developed does occur in a clearly more marked way than in the chakras described above. This is shown in an awake understanding and in intellectual skills. Scientific research conducted from a holistic point of view can also be a sign of a partially open, harmoniously functioning third eye, as well as knowledge of deep philosophical truths.

You will probably also have a well-developed faculty of visualization and intuitively capture many relationships. Your spirit is concentrated and simultaneously open to mystical truths. You become increasingly aware that the outer manifestations of things are only a simile, a symbol in which a spiritual principle is manifested on the material plane. Your thought will be carried by idealism and fantasy. You may also notice from time to time that your thoughts and ideas are fulfilled spontaneously.

The more your third eye develops, the more your thoughts will rest on direct and inner knowledge of reality. More and more people are beginning to develop partial faculties of the sixth chakra, such as clairvoyance or tactile clairvoyance on certain existential planes; others are temporarily intuitions of other dimensions of reality: for example, in meditation or in sleep.

Describing the full panoply of faculties and perceptual abilities provided by a third open eye is not possible for us. It would fill a lot of bolts and we would have to rely heavily on data provided by other people. However, here's a general overview of what awaits you with a fully developed sixth chakra.

First of all, you will perceive the world in a new way. The limits of your rational understanding will have been far exceeded. Your thinking is holographic, and you will spontaneously integrate into the knowledge process all the information that comes to you from the different fields of creation.

The material world will have become transparent to you. It is a mirror for the dance of energies that runs in the most subtle planes of creation, just as your consciousness is a mirror in which the divine being is known. Your extrasensory perception is so transparent that you will be able to directly perceive the forces that act behind the surface of the outer appearances, and you will be in a position to consciously control these energies and bring about their own forms of manifestation of these forces. But in doing so, you will be subject to certain regular laws, the framework of which you will not be able to exceed, so that natural order is preserved.

Your intuition and inner vision open the way to all the subtlest planes of reality. You know that between the plane of material creation and pure being there are infinite worlds inhabited by the most diverse essences. Before your inner eye will develop a plural drama of creation, which will seem to have no end in its ever new forms and planes of reality. A deep fear will fill you as you contemplate the greatness of this divine drama.

The most common impact of inharmonic functioning is in this case, the 'head heaviness.' You are a person who lives almost exclusively through intellect and reason. By trying to regulate everything through understanding, you only give validity to the truths that your rational thought transmits to you. Your intellectual abilities are possibly very marked and you possess the gift of shrewd analysis, but you lack the holistic vision and the ability to integrate into a great cosmic relationship.

This is how you easily come to an intellectual preponderance. You only give validity to what is grantable with understanding and verifiable, and likely with scientific methods. You reject spiritual knowledge by being scientific and unrealistic.

Also, the attempt to influence people or things with the force of thought to demonstrate one's power or to satisfy personal needs falls fully into the realm of an inharmonic functioning of the third eye. In general, the solar plexus chakra is usually altered simultaneously, and the cordial chakra and coronal will be underdeveloped. When, despite some blockages, the third eye is relatively fairly open, these attempts may also take effect, but are not in line with the natural flow of life. A sense of isolation is installed, and in the long run the satisfaction to which it is sucked is not achieved.

Another impact of misdirected energies on the sixth chakra appears when the radical chakra (and with it the "grounding") is altered, and when there are other chakras whose harmonic functioning is blocked. Then it can happen that even if you have access to the most subtle levels of perception, you do not recognize in their true significance the images and information received. These are mixed with your own ideas and fantasies, which come from your unprocessed emotional patterns. These subjectively marked images can be so dominant that you see them as the only existence, project them to the outside world and lose the reference of reality.

Hypofunction

When the flow of energies in the sixth chakra is quite clogged, for you the only reality is the visible outside world. Your life will be determined by material desires, bodily needs, and unreflective emotions. Intellectual disputes will be found stressful and useless. You reject spiritual truths, for you they are based on foolish imaginations or dreams that do not represent a practical reference. Your thinking is fundamentally oriented towards prevailing opinions.

In situations that require a lot from you, you easily lose your mind. Possibly, you're also very forgetful. Vision disturbances, which often accompany a hypofunction of the sixth chakra, are a wake-up call to look more inward and to also know those areas behind the visible surface.

In extreme cases, your thoughts can be unclear and confusing and totally determined by your unreleased emotional patterns.

Possibilities of purification and activation of the sixth chakra

Natural experience

The third eye is stimulated by the contemplation of a deeply blue night sky full of stars. This natural experience opens the spirit to the immensity and infinite depth of creation manifested with its immeasurably varied forms of manifestation, and allows to glimpse the subtle forces, structures and regular laws that execute the celestial bodies in their cosmic dance by the immensity of space, and which are also effective after the apparent manifestations of our life on Earth.

Sound therapy

Musical form: All the sounds that soothe your spirit and open it, and that evoke images and sensations of cosmic amplitude, are suitable to activate and harmonize the front chakra. Where you will most easily find the right pieces is in the music "New Age." But also some classical music from East and West, particularly Bach, can have the same effect.

Vocal: The radical chakra is activated by the vowel "i." It is sung in the key of "la" of the scale. The "i" triggers an upward-directed movement. It represents the strength of inspiration, which always leads you to new movements.

Chromotherapy

Transparent indigo affects the sixth chakra by opening and clarifying it. It gives the spirit inner tranquility, transparency and depth. In addition, it enhances and heals the senses and opens them up for more subtle planes of perception.

Gemmotherapy

Lapis lazuli: In the deep blue color of Lapis lazuli is inserted, like the stars on a night sky, golden inclusions of pyrite. It transmits to the soul an experience of security in the cosmos and opens it for infinite life in the universe. It guides the spirit inward, enhances its strength and helps you to know hierarchically superior relationships. By fostering intuition and inner vision, it allows us to recognize the hidden meaning and forces that act behind things; it also conveys a deep joy about the miracles of life and the universe.

Indigo Sapphire: A clear and transparent sapphire opens the spirit for cosmic knowledge and eternal truths. Its vibrations cause a purification, transformation and renewal of the soul and spirit. It is a bridge between the finite and the infinite, and it causes consciousness to flow along with the river of divine love and knowledge. It also gives transparency to the soul that seeks in a spiritual way.

Sodalite: The dark blue Sodalite clarifies the understanding and empowers it for deep thoughts. Its serene radiation brings serenity and strengthens nerves. Sodalite also helps to dissolve old thought patterns. It conveys confidence and strength to defend one's point of view and to transmit ideas and knowledge in everyday life.

Aromatherapy

Mint: The refreshing aroma of mint dissolves blockages in the scope of the third eye and helps to dissolve old and restrictive mental structures. It gives our spirit clarity and vivacity and promotes the strength of concentration.

Jasmine: By the subtle and outflowed scent of jasmine, our spirit opens to images and visions that carry within themselves the messages of deeper truths. Its vibrations refine perception and unite the energies of the third eye with those of the cordial chakra.

Forms of yoga that act primarily on the sixth chakra

Yoga jnana: Yoga jnana is the way of knowledge to the capacity of intellectual discernment between the real and the unreal, the eternal and the perishable. Yogi jnana knows that there is only one immutable, everlasting and eternal reality: God. In the individual's meditation, he is oriented only with the help of his power of discernment towards the absolute without attributes, to the unmanifested aspect of God, until his spirit merges with it.

Yanth Yoga: The yanths are figurative representations composed of geometric figures that symbolize the divine being and its powers and aspects. They serve as an auxiliary means for visualizations. The meditator delves into the represented aspects of divinity and patents them into its inner contemplation.

The seventh chakra and its correspondences

Keywords: Understanding, divine consciousness, cosmic consciousness, knowledge, transcendence, joy, liberation from the bonds to transcend karma. Connection with the divine mind and understanding of the functioning of the universe. You need to experience the serenity and divine joy.

- Location: At the highest part of the head.
- Sanskrit name: Sahasrara.
- Sound: None.
- Phoneme: n nasal.
- Verb: I know.
- Symbol: Lotus flower of 1,000 petals.
- Basic principle: To be pure.
- Body correspondence: Brain.
- Corresponding gland: Pineal gland (epiphysis).
- Colors: Violet, gold, and white to activate, to calm, silver and pink, better iridescent.
- Foods: Fasting.
- Essential oils: Frankincense, lotus, ylang-ylang.
- Gems: The most crystalline and pure, crystal quartz, amethyst, diamond, selenite.

The influences of epiphysis have not been fully clarified scientifically. It most likely influences the whole organism. When this gland fails, premature sexual maturity occurs.

Astrological correspondences:

- **Capricorn/Saturn:** Intuition, concentration in the essentials, penetration of matter with divine light.
- **Pisces/Neptune:** Dissolution of boundaries, delivery, unification.

CONCLUSION

The auric field is the usual name given to each person's complete energy system. It consists of seven major chakras and seven energy bodies that are in charge of assimilating the different types of energy that they nurture and that are processed in each of the levels.

This individual auric field is not a closed or isolated redoubt. It works in resonance with the environment, with other living beings, and with the Divinity. This is done in such a way that it constantly interacts by giving and taking energy and multidimensional information from the different fields that make it up. Furthermore, it also interacts with surroundings and their respective inhabitants.

Despite the differentiations, the chakras work as a team and connect with the rest of the centers. The state of harmony, known as health, is always rooted in the harmonic balance of the openings and expressions that occur in the seven main centers. Having one chakra very open and another functioning half-closed produces a distortion that inevitably leads to disharmony and brings problems in some areas of life.

By paying due attention to your energy state, you can begin to improve the control of the chakras, using different tools that are easily accessible to improve our general state and begin to enjoy harmony.

Achieving harmony in our life is no-nonsense. The balance between everything we are, everything we have and everything we want to achieve is essential to have optimal well-being. And how could it be otherwise? To find order and peace in our life, we first have to find it in ourselves. The chakras are the energy centers of our body, a kind of door through which energy flows. A decompensation of our chakras can bring fatal consequences since it produces an imbalance between our energy which causes us to go into crisis.